TAI CHI WALKING FOR SENIORS

A Step-by-Step Guide to Improve Balance, Prevent Falls, and Soothe Joint Stiffness

MARIAN COLEWOOD

Table Of Content

Introduction

The Path to Lifelong Stability

You might know the feeling all too well. You wake up in the morning, and before you even get out of bed, you do a mental check-in. How are the knees today? Is the lower back stiff? When you stand up, you might take a moment to steady yourself, waiting for that feeling of stability to kick in before you take your first step.

For many of us, as we age, walking—the most natural human movement—changes. It stops being something we do automatically and starts becoming something we have to manage. You might find yourself looking at the ground more often to avoid tripping. You might hesitate before stepping off a curb. Or perhaps you simply walk less because the "good kind of tired" you used to feel after exercise has been replaced by the "bad kind of pain" in your joints.

This hesitation often leads to a vicious cycle: we move less to avoid pain or falls, but moving less actually makes us stiffer and *more* prone to falling.

It is time to break that cycle.

This book is not about training for a marathon, and it isn't about complex martial arts routines that require you to memorize fifty different moves. It is about taking the activity you do every day—walking—and transforming it into a tool for healing, strength, and confidence.

The Myth of "I'm Too Old"

There is a pervasive myth that losing your balance and mobility is an inevitable part of aging. While it is true that our bodies change—our reaction times slow down and our joints may lose some cushioning—losing your independence is not a guarantee.

The human body is incredibly adaptable. Even in your 60s, 70s, 80s, and beyond, your muscles can get stronger, and your nervous system can learn new patterns. The problem isn't usually *age*; the problem is *mechanics*.

Most people spend their lives "falling forward" when they walk. They lean their upper body ahead of their feet and rely on momentum to catch them. When you are young, you can get away with this. When you are older, this habit becomes dangerous.

Why Tai Chi Walking?

Tai Chi Walking is different. It is often described as "meditation in motion," but don't let the spiritual sounding name fool you—it is deeply grounded in biomechanics.

Unlike regular walking, where you fall onto your foot, Tai Chi Walking teaches you to **place** your foot. It teaches you how to shift 100% of your weight securely onto one leg before you even lift the other. It teaches you to keep your knees soft to absorb shock, rather than locking them and jarring your hips and spine.

It turns a frantic, unconscious stumble into a deliberate, powerful stride.

The Triple Benefit

In this book, we will focus on three specific outcomes. These are the pillars of your physical independence:

1. Improving Balance: You will learn to control your center of gravity. By the end of this book, you won't just hope you don't fall; you will trust your legs to hold you up.
2. Preventing Falls: Falls often happen during the transition between steps. We will slow that transition

down, strengthening the stabilizer muscles that catch you when you trip.

3. Soothing Joint Stiffness: Motion is lotion. The gentle, rhythmic nature of this walking style pumps synovial fluid into your joints, reducing the "creakiness" of arthritis and inactivity without the high impact of jogging or aerobics.

How to Use This Book

This is a practical manual. We have titled it a "Step-by-Step Guide" because that is exactly how you should treat it. You do not need special equipment, a gym membership, or a large studio. You only need a small hallway, a living room, or a quiet path in the park.

We will start by assessing where you are today. Then, we will look at the foundation: your posture and your breathing. Finally, we will learn the walk itself, breaking it down into manageable pieces so you never feel overwhelmed.

Your journey to better mobility doesn't require a giant leap. It begins with a single, mindful step. Let's take that step together.

PART 1

THE FOUNDATION– PREPARING BODY AND MIND

Chapter 1

Assessing Your Starting Point

The journey toward improved mobility and confidence begins not with a single step forward, but with a pause to understand where the body stands in the present moment. Before attempting to master the fluid movements of Tai Chi walking, an honest and thorough assessment of current capabilities is essential. This process is not about judging physical limitations or lamenting the changes that come with age; rather, it is about creating a precise map of the starting terrain. Just as a builder must survey the land before laying a foundation, an individual must understand the unique quirks, strengths, and vulnerabilities of their own physiology. This baseline knowledge ensures that every subsequent exercise is safe, effective, and tailored to specific needs. By establishing a clear starting point, progress becomes measurable, and the fear of the unknown—often the root cause of anxiety regarding falls—is replaced by the certainty of self-knowledge.

Simple self-tests to check your current balance and range of motion

Establishing a baseline for balance and flexibility does not require expensive medical equipment or a visit to a specialist; it can be accomplished effectively in the safety of a living room using simple, functional movements. However, safety must remain the paramount concern during this assessment phase. A sturdy chair or a kitchen counter should always be within arm's reach to provide support if steadiness falters. The first area of evaluation is static balance, which reveals how well the body maintains stability when stationary. A fundamental method for testing this is the Romberg Test, adapted for home use. The individual stands with feet together, ankles touching, and arms crossed over the chest. The goal is to hold this position for thirty seconds with eyes open. This simple stance forces the body to rely on proprioception—the internal sense of body position—rather than a wide base of support. If this feels stable, the challenge increases by closing the eyes. Removing visual input forces the brain to rely entirely on the inner ear and the sensory nerves in the feet to maintain an upright position. Swaying slightly is normal, but a need to step out or grab a support indicates that the vestibular system or foot sensitivity may need specific attention during the training to come.

Following the static assessment, dynamic balance must be evaluated, as this is the type of balance required for walking. The Tandem Stance test provides excellent insight here. This involves placing one foot directly in front of the other, heel to toe, like standing on a tightrope. This position creates a narrow base of support that mimics the critical transition phase of walking where weight transfers from one leg to the other. Holding this pose for ten to fifteen seconds on each side reveals asymmetries; often, an individual will discover that one leg is significantly more stable than the other. This discrepancy is vital information, as most falls occur on the "weak side" during a moment of distraction. Recognizing which leg offers less stability allows for targeted practice during the Tai Chi walking drills that will follow in later chapters.

Beyond balance, the range of motion in the lower body dictates the fluidity of the stride. Stiffness in the ankles is a primary contributor to tripping, as a foot that cannot flex upward (dorsiflexion) is more likely to catch on rugs or uneven pavement. To test ankle flexibility, one can sit in a chair and attempt to keep the heel on the ground while lifting the toes as high as possible. If the foot barely clears the floor, or if the movement causes strain in the shin, ankle stiffness is likely present. Similarly, hip mobility plays a crucial role. While standing and holding a support, lifting one knee toward the chest as high as comfort allows demonstrates the hip's capacity for flexion. If the knee cannot rise to hip height without the upper body leaning backward to compensate, the hip flexors are tight. This tightness forces a shorter, shuffling stride that reduces stability. These self-tests act as diagnostic tools, highlighting exactly which "hinges" of the body need lubrication and which muscles need awakening.

Identifying "danger zones" in your daily movement patterns

Once the physical baseline is established, the focus must shift to the behavioral and environmental factors that contribute to instability. These are the "danger zones"—habits and surroundings that increase the risk of falling regardless of physical strength. Identifying these zones requires a high degree of mindfulness and an objective look at daily routines. The most treacherous danger zones are often behavioral, rooted in the subconscious habits developed over a lifetime. The "rush reflex" is a prime example. When the phone rings, the doorbell chimes, or a timer goes off in the kitchen, the instinct is to move immediately and quickly. For a senior body that requires a moment to calibrate blood pressure and balance upon standing, this sudden burst of movement is a common cause of dizziness and subsequent falls. Recognizing this tendency allows an individual to consciously pause, take a breath, and engage the muscles before moving, overriding the reactive impulse with a safe, deliberate action.

Another critical behavioral danger zone is the transition between different types of movements or surfaces. Moving from a seated position to a standing position is biomechanically complex, requiring a shift in the center of gravity and a burst of leg strength. Many individuals unconsciously hold their breath during this exertion, which can deprive the brain of oxygen and cause momentary lightheadedness. Similarly, transitioning from a carpeted living room to a tiled kitchen changes the friction underfoot instantly. A stride that is safe on carpet might lead to a slip on smooth tile. Assessing how one navigates these transitions is crucial. Does the individual look down at the floor while walking? While this seems like a safety precaution to spot obstacles, it actually shifts the center of gravity forward and strains the neck, throwing off the body's natural alignment. The ideal gaze is forward, scanning the environment, rather than fixed directly on the toes.

Environmental danger zones within the home also demand a critical audit. This goes beyond simply removing loose rugs. It involves analyzing the lighting in hallways and stairwells, as shadows can distort depth perception and hide obstacles. It involves checking the footwear worn inside the house. Socks on a wooden floor or loose-fitting slippers that do not cup the heel are significant hazards. A common but often overlooked danger zone is the "clutter of convenience"—objects placed on stairs to be carried up later, or cords stretched across walkways for easy access to electronics. By systematically observing where hesitation or stumbling occurs during the day—perhaps a specific turn in the hallway or a difficult step down into the garage—one identifies the specific environments that require the application of Tai Chi walking principles. These zones are not necessarily places to avoid, but rather places where focus must be sharpened and technique applied with rigor.

Setting realistic goals: From walking to the mailbox to walking the park loop

With a clear understanding of physical capabilities and environmental challenges, the final step in the preparation phase is the establishment of concrete, achievable goals. Motivation often burns out when ambition outpaces ability. Setting goals that are too lofty too soon can lead to frustration, pain, or injury, which reinforces the cycle of inactivity. Therefore, the goal-setting process must be gradual, celebrating small victories that compound over time into significant life changes. The progression should be viewed as a ladder, where each rung must be secure before stepping up to the next.

The first tier of goals should be purely functional and rooted in the immediate surroundings. For someone who has been sedentary or struggling with fear of falling, the initial goal might be as simple as "walking to the mailbox and back with zero hesitation." This objective is specific and measurable. It does not focus on distance or speed, but on the *quality* of the movement. The aim is to apply the breathing and weight-shifting techniques learned in this book to a short, familiar route. Achieving this creates a psychological win. It proves that control is possible. Once the mailbox run becomes routine and comfortable, the goalpost moves.

The intermediate tier involves extending endurance and navigating more complex environments. A "block walk" or a visit to a local store introduces variables like uneven sidewalks, other pedestrians, and traffic signals. Here, the goal shifts from simple execution to consistency and adaptability. A realistic target might be "walking for fifteen minutes continuously without stopping to rest." This builds cardiovascular health alongside balance. It is important to measure this progress not just by the clock, but by the body's feedback. Using a Rate of Perceived Exertion (RPE) scale—where 1 is sitting on the couch and 10 is sprinting uphill—helps in regulating effort. The target for Tai Chi walking is a moderate 3 or 4, where breathing is deeper but conversation is still possible.

The long-term aspiration, the "Park Loop," represents the culmination of physical conditioning and confidence. A park loop often involves changing elevations, grass, gravel, and distractions like dogs or children. Navigating this environment successfully signifies that the principles of balance and stability have become second nature. However, reaching this stage requires patience. It is vital to understand that progress is rarely linear. There will be days of stiffness and days of high energy. Listening to the body is part of the discipline. If a "bad knee day" occurs, the goal adjusts to a gentle indoor session rather than forcing a park walk. This flexibility prevents setbacks.

Ultimately, the purpose of setting these goals is to shift the mindset from "avoiding falls" to "cultivating freedom." The objective is not just to prevent an accident, but to regain the ability to say "yes" to life's invitations—whether that is a stroll with a grandchild, a shopping trip, or simply enjoying the fresh air. By grounding aspirations in reality and building them step-by-step, the path to mobility becomes a rewarding journey of self-discovery rather than a grueling regime of exercise. The transformation happens not in the destination, but in the confidence gained with every mindful, stable step taken along the way.

Chapter 2

Safety First – Gear and Environment

The transition from intent to action requires a bridge, and that bridge is constructed of preparation. Before a single step of Tai Chi walking is taken, the external and internal conditions must be optimized to ensure that the practice builds strength rather than inviting injury. Safety is not merely about avoiding accidents; it is about creating a psychological and physical container where confidence can flourish. When the fear of slipping or tripping is removed through deliberate preparation, the mind is free to focus on the subtleties of movement, breath, and balance. This chapter explores the essential equipment—specifically footwear—and the environmental factors that transform a simple room or garden into a sanctuary of stability. Furthermore, it delves into the crucial skill of interpreting the body's sensory feedback, establishing a new language of communication between physical sensation and conscious awareness.

Footwear Essentials: Choosing shoes that support stability without restricting movement

The foot is an engineering marvel, a complex structure of twenty-six bones, thirty-three joints, and over one hundred muscles, tendons, and ligaments designed to absorb shock and provide propulsion. In the context of Tai Chi walking, the foot acts as the primary sensor, gathering data about the ground—its texture, slope, and stability—and transmitting that information to the brain. This continuous feedback loop, known as proprioception, is the cornerstone of balance. Therefore, the choice of footwear is not merely a matter of fashion or even standard comfort; it is a matter of maintaining the fidelity of this sensory transmission. A shoe that is too thick, too rigid, or poorly fitted acts as a blindfold for the feet, dampening the vital signals required to stay upright.

Selecting the correct shoe involves finding a delicate balance between protection and sensitivity. Modern athletic shoes often prioritize maximal cushioning, featuring thick, cloud-like soles that completely isolate the foot from the ground. While this may feel pleasant while standing still, it can be detrimental during the mindful movement of Tai Chi walking. A sole that is too soft creates instability, much like trying to balance on a mattress. The foot struggles to find a solid reference point, forcing the ankles and knees to work overtime to maintain equilibrium. The ideal shoe for this practice features a firm, low-profile sole that offers enough protection to prevent bruising from pebbles or hard surfaces while remaining thin enough to allow the wearer to feel the floor. This "ground feel" is essential for the weight-shifting mechanics discussed later in the book. The practitioner needs to sense exactly when the weight has fully transferred to the heel, the ball of the foot, and the toes.

Another critical feature to scrutinize is the heel drop, which refers to the difference in height between the heel and the toe. Traditional running shoes and even many walking shoes elevate the heel significantly, tipping the body's center of gravity forward. For a senior seeking stability, this forward tilt is counterproductive, as it shortens the calf muscles and destabilizes the posture. A "zero-drop" or low-drop shoe, where the heel and toe are at roughly the same level, encourages a more natural, upright alignment. This flat platform mimics the biomechanics of being barefoot, allowing the Achilles tendon to lengthen and the spine to stack naturally over the hips. When the skeleton is properly aligned, the muscles do not have to strain to hold the body up, reducing fatigue and the risk of back pain.

The construction of the toe box is equally important. Many fashion-forward shoes taper at the front, squeezing the toes together. However, for maximum stability, the toes need to splay—spread out wide—upon contact with the ground. This splaying action increases the surface area of the base of support, acting like the roots of a tree anchoring into the earth. A shoe with a wide, anatomical toe box allows the big toe to function as a stabilizer. If the toes are compressed, balance is compromised laterally. The material of the upper shoe should be breathable and flexible, moving with the foot rather than acting as a cast. Stiff leather or rigid plastics can restrict the natural flexion of the metatarsals, leading to a clunky, robotic gait rather than the smooth, rolling motion required for Tai Chi walking.

The method of securing the shoe to the foot also warrants attention. Slip-on shoes, while convenient, often lack the structural integrity to hold the heel firmly in place. If the heel slides up and down inside the shoe, the toes will instinctively claw downward to grip the sole, creating tension in the arch and shin. Laces or adjustable Velcro straps are superior because they allow for a customized fit that locks the heel into the "heel cup" of the shoe. This security ensures that the shoe moves as an extension of the foot, rather than an external object that must be dragged along. When trying on shoes, it is advisable to do so in the late afternoon, as feet tend to swell slightly throughout the day. A shoe that fits perfectly in the morning may become restrictively tight by evening. The correct fit should allow for a thumb's width of space between the longest toe and the front of the shoe, ensuring that there is no impingement even during the push-off phase of the stride.

The Practice Space: Creating a hazard-free zone in your living room or garden

Once the foundation of footwear is secured, attention must turn to the environment in which the practice will take place. The ideal practice space is not necessarily a professional studio or a vast expanse of land; it is simply a controlled environment where hazards have been systematically identified and neutralized. This process of "hazard-proofing" is a critical step in fall prevention. The living room is often the most convenient location, but it is frequently filled with obstacles that become invisible through familiarity. The first enemy of safe movement in the home is the throw rug. While aesthetically pleasing, unsecured rugs are the leading cause of in-home falls. The edges can curl up, or the rug can slide underfoot during a weight shift. For the purpose of Tai Chi walking, the practice area must be cleared of all loose floor coverings. The surface should be consistent—either bare wood, laminate, or wall-to-wall carpeting.

Transitions between different floor types should be avoided within the immediate practice zone to maintain a predictable friction coefficient.

Lighting plays a surprisingly vital role in balance. As vision changes with age, the need for bright, even illumination increases. Dim lighting or harsh shadows can distort depth perception, making a flat floor appear uneven or hiding small objects. The practice space should be well-lit, ideally with natural light or bright, diffuse overhead lighting. Glare from polished floors or direct sunlight hitting a window can be disorienting, so the use of sheer curtains or adjusting the angle of blinds is recommended. The visual field should also be relatively uncluttered. A space packed with furniture, patterned wallpapers, and scattered objects can be visually noisy, taxing the brain as it tries to process spatial orientation. Creating a "visual anchor"—a clear, steady point to focus on at eye level—helps stabilize the body during movement. This could be a picture on the wall or a specific tree in the garden.

Space requirements for Tai Chi walking are modest, but specific. The practitioner needs enough room to take three to four strides in a straight line and enough width to extend the arms fully without hitting furniture or walls. This "buffer zone" is crucial for psychological safety. If the mind is subconsciously worried about knocking over a vase or hitting a sharp table corner, the body will tighten up, restricting the fluidity of the movement. A clear path of roughly six feet by four feet is usually sufficient. If space is limited, the practice can be adapted to a smaller footprint, but the area must be strictly dedicated to the movement during the session. Pets, while beloved companions, introduce an element of unpredictability. During practice, dogs and cats should be secured in another room to prevent them from weaving between legs or creating sudden distractions.

For those who prefer to practice outdoors, the garden or a local park offers fresh air and a connection to nature, but these environments introduce new variables. The ground must be inspected for flatness. A lawn might hide small divots, tree roots, or patches of soft mud that can twist an ankle. Concrete or paved patios offer stability but are unforgiving if a stumble occurs. Beginners should start on firm, level surfaces like a paved driveway or a tennis court before graduating to grass. Wind is another factor; a strong gust can affect balance, especially when standing on one leg. Awareness of the weather conditions is part of the safety protocol. Wet leaves, morning dew on grass, or patches of moss can be as slippery as ice. The outdoor practitioner must be vigilant, scanning the "terrain" before beginning the walk, ensuring that the chosen path is free of loose gravel or debris that could act like ball bearings under the shoe.

The auditory environment also contributes to safety. While music can be relaxing, it can sometimes mask the sound of one's own footsteps or breathing, which are important feedback mechanisms. Practicing in relative silence, or with very soft, consistent background noise, allows for greater concentration. Sudden loud noises—a slamming door, a car backfiring—can trigger the "startle reflex," causing the muscles to jerk and potentially destabilizing the posture. Creating a quiet zone helps maintain the calm, parasympathetic nervous system state that is conducive to learning and balance. If practicing in a public park, finding a spot away from active sports fields or busy playgrounds minimizes the risk of collision or distraction. The goal is to create a "bubble" of protected space where the external world recedes, allowing the internal world of movement to take center stage.

Listening to the Body: Distinguishing between "good" effort and "bad" pain signals

The final and perhaps most profound aspect of safety is the internal dialogue between the mind and the body. In a culture that often glorifies the mantra "no pain, no gain," learning to discern the nuances of physical sensation is a radical act of self-preservation. For the senior practitioner, the "no pain, no gain" philosophy is not only outdated but dangerous. Pain is the body's alarm system, a high-priority signal that tissue damage is imminent or occurring. Ignoring this signal in favor of pushing through a barrier can lead to setbacks that take months to heal. However, fear of any sensation can lead to paralysis and atrophy. The key is to learn the difference between the "discomfort of growth" and the "pain of injury."

"Good" effort has distinct characteristics. It is often felt as a dull, generalized warmth in the muscles, particularly in the thighs and glutes. This sensation is the feeling of muscle fibers engaging and working. It may be accompanied by a slight burning sensation that dissipates quickly once the movement stops or the intensity is reduced. This is the feeling of strength building. Another form of good sensation is the feeling of stretching or tension in tight areas, such as the hips or calves. This "sweet pain" feels satisfying, like an itch being scratched. It is a sign that shortened tissues are being lengthened. Crucially, good effort leaves the practitioner feeling energized and looser after the session, even if there is some mild fatigue. The breath may quicken, and the heart rate may rise, but these should remain within a comfortable range where conversation is still possible.

"Bad" pain, conversely, speaks a different language. It is often sharp, stabbing, or shooting in nature. It tends to be highly localized—a specific point in the knee, a pinch in the lower back, or a sharp twinge in the ankle. This type of pain often feels "wrong" instinctively. Sensations that feel electrical or like a sudden jolt are warning signs of nerve impingement and should result in an immediate cessation of the movement. Joint pain that feels like grinding, clicking with pain, or a deep ache within the bone is a signal to stop. Unlike muscle fatigue, which resolves with rest, bad pain often lingers or worsens hours after the practice has ended. Swelling, redness, or heat around a joint are inflammatory responses that demand rest and ice, not further movement.

A fundamental principle to navigate this territory is the "70% Rule." This concept advises that one should never perform a movement to their absolute maximum capacity. If a knee can bend to 90 degrees, the practitioner should only bend it to roughly 70 degrees during the practice. By staying within this buffer zone, the body remains relaxed and fluid. When pushed to 100% of capacity, the muscles tense up in a protective reflex, bracing against the limit. This tension blocks the flow of movement and increases the risk of strain. By working at 70%, the body learns to trust the movement, and over time, the 70% limit naturally expands. What was once a limit becomes easy, and the range of motion increases without force. This approach prioritizes longevity over intensity.

It is also vital to recognize systemic warning signs that go beyond musculoskeletal pain. Dizziness, lightheadedness, or seeing spots are signs that the blood pressure has dropped or the brain is not receiving enough oxygen. This is not a signal to "push through"; it is a command to sit down immediately. Nausea, cold sweats, or chest pressure are medical red flags that require immediate attention. The practitioner must also be attuned to the "delayed onset" signals. Sometimes, a session feels fine in the moment, but pain appears the next morning. This indicates that the volume or intensity of the practice was too high. The remedy is not to quit, but to scale back the duration or depth of the movements in the next session. Listening to the body is a skill that improves with practice. It requires honesty and the humility to accept that the body's needs change from day to day. One day, a twenty-minute walk feels effortless; the next day, ten minutes may be the limit. Respecting these fluctuations is the hallmark of an advanced practitioner. By honoring the body's signals, the practitioner ensures that they can return to the practice day after day, building a cumulative effect of strength and stability that lasts a lifetime.

Chapter 3

The Pillars of Posture

The human body is an architectural marvel, a structure designed to resist gravity while allowing for fluid, dynamic motion. However, over decades of life, gravity often claims a slow victory, compressing the spine, rounding the shoulders, and stiffening the joints. This gradual collapse is not merely an aesthetic concern; it is the primary culprit behind chronic pain, diminished energy, and the loss of balance. To master Tai Chi walking, the practitioner must first rebuild the internal structure. This does not require building massive muscles, but rather realigning the skeletal frame so that the bones, not the muscles, bear the weight of the body. When the skeleton is stacked correctly, muscular tension melts away, and the body becomes a conduit for energy rather than a heavy burden to be dragged around. This chapter explores the three non-negotiable pillars of this alignment: the suspension of the head, the relaxation of the chest, and the softening of the knees. Together, these elements transform the body from a rigid, fragile object into a resilient, adaptable system.

The "Suspended Head": Aligning the spine to reduce back pain

The head is a significant weight, averaging between ten and twelve pounds—roughly the weight of a bowling ball. When this weight sits perfectly atop the cervical spine, the neck muscles have very little work to do. However, in modern daily life, the head often migrates forward. Years of looking down at books, working at computers, or simply peering at the ground to avoid tripping creates a postural habit known as "forward head carriage." For every inch the head moves forward past the shoulders, the effective weight on the neck muscles doubles. This leverage places immense strain not only on the cervical vertebrae but on the entire spinal chain. The body is a continuous tensegrity structure; tension in the neck pulls on the upper back, which in turn distorts the lumbar curve, leading to chronic lower back pain. Therefore, the first step in Tai Chi walking is to reclaim the vertical axis by "suspending" the head.

The ancient Tai Chi classics describe this principle as Xu Ling Ding Jin, which translates to "an intangible energy lifting the crown of the head." The practitioner should imagine a golden thread attached to the very top of the skull—specifically the crown point, or Bai Hui—gently pulling upward toward the sky. This visualization is crucial because it engages the deep postural muscles without creating rigidity. It is not a military command to "stand tall," which usually results in a stiff, arched back and a lifted chin. Instead, it is a subtle, internal elongation. Imagine the spine as a string of pearls resting on a table. If one pushes the pearls from the bottom, the string buckles and twists. But if one gently pulls the string from the top, the pearls naturally align into a straight, fluid line. This is the effect of the suspended head. It creates space between the vertebrae, allowing the intervertebral discs to hydrate and decompreess, offering immediate relief to a spine that has been compacted by gravity.

A critical component of this suspension is the position of the chin. When the head is pulled upward, there is a natural tendency to lift the chin, but this actually compresses the back of the neck. To achieve the correct alignment, the chin must be slightly tucked, as if holding a small peach between the chin and the throat. This action flattens the cervical curve, lengthening the back of the neck and opening the base of the skull where the spine meets the brainstem. This area, the occipital ridge, is a common reservoir for tension headaches and dizziness. By lengthening this region, the practitioner opens the neural pathways, improving the communication between the brain and the body. The sensation should be one of the back of the neck lengthening upward while the face relaxes downward.

This alignment also plays a pivotal role in balance. The vestibular system, located in the inner ear, is the body's internal gyroscope. It tells the brain where the body is in space. If the head is habitually tilted forward or cocked to one side, the gyroscope is calibrated incorrectly. The brain receives skewed data, making the practitioner feel unsteady. By leveling the head and suspending the crown, the inner ear is brought into a neutral, optimal position. The eyes, too, are affected. With the head suspended, the gaze naturally settles on the horizon rather than the feet. This horizon-gaze is essential for stability. Looking down shifts the center of gravity forward, inviting a fall. Looking straight ahead keeps the weight centered over the arches of the feet. The suspended head serves as the "North Star" of the body's navigation system; when it is true, the rest of the body can organize itself around that vertical line with minimal effort.

Sinking the Chest, Raising the Back: Relieving tension in the upper body

While the head reaches for the sky, the upper torso must learn to settle downward. This principle is often the most counterintuitive for Western practitioners who have been raised on the instruction to "stand up straight, chest out, shoulders back." The military posture of puffing out the chest is detrimental to stability and relaxation. When the chest is thrust forward, the thoracic spine locks into a rigid extension, the lower back sways excessively (lordosis), and the center of gravity rises. A high center of gravity makes the body top-heavy and unstable, like an inverted pyramid. Furthermore, puffing the chest restricts the movement of the diaphragm. It locks the breath in the upper chest, leading to shallow, anxious breathing that triggers the sympathetic nervous system—the fight-or-flight response. To find calm and stability, the practitioner must learn to "sink" the chest.

Sinking the chest, or Han Xiong, does not mean slouching or collapsing the structure. It is not a depressive posture where the shoulders roll forward and the head droops. Rather, it is an internal softening of the sternum. The practitioner should imagine that the breastbone is made of soft wax melting slightly under the warmth of the sun. As the sternum softens and moves slightly inward, the ribs relax, allowing the breath to sink deep into the belly. This action protects the heart and lungs, creating a sensation of containment and safety. It acts as a shield. Biomechanically, this softening allows the shoulder blades to slide apart slightly, broadening the upper back. This is the second half of the principle: "Raising the Back," or Ba Bei.

Raising the back refers to the subtle rounding and expansion of the area between the shoulder blades. Imagine the back is like the shell of a tortoise—rounded, strong, and protective. When the chest sinks and the back rounds slightly, the spine assumes a "bow" shape. This is a structure of immense strength. A straight rod is brittle and easily broken, but a bow can absorb force and spring back. By adopting this subtle curve, the upper body becomes capable of absorbing the shock of walking without jarring the neck or head. It connects the arms to the spine, integrating the upper body into a single, unified unit. This structure is essential for balance recovery. If a person with a rigid, puffed chest stumbles, their upper body acts as a stiff lever, throwing them off balance further. A person with a sunk chest and rounded back has the flexibility to absorb the stumble and recover.

This posture also has a profound effect on emotional regulation. Physical tension in the chest is often the somatic storage site for anxiety and grief. By consciously softening this area, the practitioner sends a signal to the vagus nerve that it is safe to relax. The breath drops from the clavicles down to the abdomen, lowering the heart rate and blood pressure. The shoulders, which often creep up toward the ears in response to stress, naturally drop down. The instruction "shoulders down" is often ineffective if the chest is puffed; the anatomy forces the shoulders up. But the moment the chest sinks, the shoulders have no choice but to slide down the back, guided by gravity. This releases the chronic tension in the trapezius muscles that plagues so many seniors.

The dynamic relationship between the suspended head and the sunk chest creates a vertical stretch. The neck pulls up, the shoulders sink down. This two-way stretch opens the thoracic outlet, improving circulation to the arms and hands. Many practitioners report a sensation of warmth or tingling in the fingers—a sign that blood flow, previously restricted by tight shoulders, has been restored. Sinking the chest essentially "seats" the upper body onto the lower body, connecting the torso to the hips. It ensures that when the legs move, the upper body follows smoothly, rather than lagging behind or tipping forward. It is the physical embodiment of composure.

Soft Knees: The secret to protecting joints and absorbing shock

The foundation of the entire Tai Chi walking structure lies in the knees. They are the shock absorbers of the body, the mechanism that mediates the relationship between the heavy torso and the unyielding ground. Yet, the knee is often the site of greatest pain and vulnerability for seniors. The instinct, when standing or walking, is often to lock the legs straight. This locking provides a false sense of skeletal stability—it feels easier to stack the bones than to use the muscles. However, a locked knee is a disaster for mobility. When the leg is straight and the joint is locked, the flow of circulation is pinched off. More critically, a locked leg cannot absorb shock. Every step sends a jarring impact up the tibia, straight through the locked knee, and into the hip and lower back. Over thousands of steps a day, this micro-trauma grinds down cartilage and inflames the joints.

To "soften" the knees does not mean walking in a deep crouch or a squat, which would be exhausting and damaging. It refers to a state of "unlocked readiness." The leg should never be fully straight, even when it is the weight-bearing leg. There should always be a micro-bend, a slight flexion that keeps the muscles of the thigh (quadriceps) and the back of the leg (hamstrings) gently engaged. Imagine standing on a boat that is rocking gently on the waves. Instinctively, one would bend the knees to lower the center of gravity and absorb the motion of the boat. This is the "soft knee" state. It lowers the body's center of mass, instantly increasing stability. A lower center of gravity is like the ballast in a ship; it makes the practitioner harder to topple.

This softness allows for fluid weight transfer. In Tai Chi walking, the transition of weight from one foot to the other must be seamless, like sand pouring from an hourglass. If the knee is locked, the weight "clunks" onto the leg. If the knee is soft, it acts as a spring, compressing gently to accept the weight and then extending to push the body forward. This spring-like action pumps fluid through the joint capsule. Cartilage has no blood supply; it relies on the compression and release of movement to absorb nutrients from the synovial fluid. Therefore, walking with soft knees is not just safer; it is therapeutic. It actively feeds the knee joint, helping to repair and maintain the cushioning surfaces.

Maintaining soft knees also unlocks the hips. The body is a kinetic chain; what happens at the knee affects the hip. A locked knee forces the hip to hike up, creating unevenness in the pelvis and strain in the lower back. A soft knee allows the femoral head to rotate freely in the hip socket. This rotation is crucial for turning and changing direction. For seniors, the inability to pivot quickly is a major cause of falls. When the knees are supple, the body can pivot on the heel or the ball of the foot with ease. When they are locked, a turn creates torque, twisting the knee joint and risking ligament damage.

The mental component of soft knees is a feeling of "rooting." The practitioner should imagine that, through the relaxed joints of the legs, their weight is sinking deep into the earth, like the roots of an old oak tree. This connection to the ground provides a psychological anchor. When the knees are locked, the energy feels stuck in the head, leading to top-heaviness and anxiety. When the knees soften, the energy drops. The practitioner feels "grounded." This is not just a metaphor; physically, the contact surface of the foot engages more completely with the floor when the knees are bent. The toes can spread, and the arch can activate.

Developing the strength to maintain this soft bend takes time. Initially, the thigh muscles may feel warm or tired, as they are being asked to support the body in a way they haven't in years. This is positive feedback. It indicates that the burden of gravity is being shifted from the passive joints to the active muscles. Strong quadriceps are the best insurance policy for knee health. By consistently practicing with soft knees—while brushing teeth, waiting in line, or washing dishes—the practitioner builds the muscular endurance required for longer walks. Eventually, the locked-leg habit is overwritten, and the soft, springy, resilient gait of Tai Chi walking becomes the new normal, protecting the skeleton with every step.

PART 2

THE MECHANICS – MASTERING THE MOVEMENT

Chapter 4

The Engine of Breath

Movement without breath is merely physical exertion, but movement synchronized with breath becomes a source of revitalization and internal power. In the practice of Tai Chi walking, the breath serves as the engine that drives the vehicle of the body. It dictates the rhythm, provides the fuel for muscular endurance, and acts as the bridge between the conscious mind and the physiological systems. For the senior practitioner, mastering the breath is often more critical than mastering the footwork. As the body ages, lung capacity naturally diminishes, and the ribcage can become rigid, leading to shallow, inefficient respiration. This chapter focuses on reclaiming the full capacity of the lungs, transforming the act of breathing from a subconscious survival mechanism into a deliberate tool for stability, health, and pain management.

Diaphragmatic breathing techniques to oxygenate muscles and calm the nervous system

Most adults, over the course of a lifetime, develop a habit of shallow chest breathing. This type of respiration, often driven by stress or poor posture, utilizes only the upper lobes of the lungs. When a person breathes into the chest, the shoulders rise, the neck muscles tense, and the gas exchange is minimal. This signals the sympathetic nervous system—the "fight or flight" response—that the body is in danger, flooding the bloodstream with cortisol and adrenaline. For a senior seeking balance and calm, this state of chronic low-level stress is counterproductive. It creates muscle tension that restricts range of motion and heightens the perception of pain. The antidote to this condition is diaphragmatic breathing, often referred to as "belly breathing" or "kidney breathing" in internal arts.

The diaphragm is a large, dome-shaped muscle located at the base of the ribcage, separating the chest cavity from the abdominal cavity. In proper breathing, the diaphragm contracts and moves downward during inhalation. This downward movement creates a vacuum that pulls air deep into the bottom of the lungs, where the majority of blood vessels are located. This maximizes oxygen exchange, delivering a richer supply of nutrients to the brain and muscles. As the diaphragm descends, it physically pushes the abdominal organs downward and outward, causing the belly to expand. This is why it is called belly breathing. It is not that air is entering the stomach, but that the mechanics of the lung expansion are displacing the internal organs. This gentle internal massage improves digestion and circulation within the abdominal cavity, addressing common issues like constipation or sluggish metabolism often found in older adults.

To learn this technique, the practitioner should begin in a seated or lying position where gravity does not challenge the posture. Placing one hand on the chest and one hand on the belly provides tactile feedback. The goal is to inhale slowly through the nose, directing the air "down" toward the navel. The hand on the belly should rise, while the hand on the chest remains relatively still. If the chest hand rises, the breath is too shallow. The visualization of filling a balloon is helpful here; a balloon fills from the bottom up. Similarly, the lungs should fill from the base, expanding the lower ribs laterally and the abdomen anteriorly. This requires a conscious relaxation of the abdominal muscles. Many people hold their stomachs in due to vanity or tension; this "sucking in" paralyzes the diaphragm. To breathe well, one must let the belly go soft.

The physiological impact of this technique extends far beyond oxygenation. The diaphragm is intimately connected to the vagus nerve, the longest nerve of the autonomic nervous system. The vagus nerve acts as the brake pedal for the body's stress response. Deep, rhythmic diaphragmatic breathing stimulates this nerve, triggering the parasympathetic nervous system—the "rest and digest" state. This creates an immediate physiological cascade: heart rate slows, blood pressure drops, and muscle tension dissipates. For a senior about to embark on a walk, this pre-exercise calming is vital. It reduces the "performance anxiety" associated with fear of falling. When the nervous system is calm, proprioception (the sense of body position) improves, and the brain can process balance information more accurately.

Furthermore, diaphragmatic breathing creates internal pressure—intra-abdominal pressure—that stabilizes the spine. Imagine an unopened soda can; the pressure inside makes the thin aluminum walls incredibly strong and able to support weight. When one breathes deep into the belly, it pressurizes the core, creating a pillar of air that supports the lumbar spine from the inside out. This pneumatic support reduces the load on the back muscles and vertebral discs. Therefore, every deep breath is not just an intake of air; it is a momentary act of spinal traction and stabilization. Mastering this breath while stationary is the prerequisite for moving. The practitioner must condition the body to default to this deep, rhythmic pattern, ensuring that even when the physical demand of walking increases, the breath remains the anchor of stability.

Coordinating breath with movement: Inhale to prepare, exhale to move

Once the diaphragm is engaged, the next challenge is to synchronize this respiratory rhythm with physical motion. In ordinary walking, breathing is often erratic or disconnected from the stride. In Tai Chi walking, the breath and the step are locked in a harmonious dance. This coordination serves a biomechanical purpose: it ensures that the body is most stable when the breath is leaving, and most receptive when the breath is entering. The fundamental rule to follow is simple yet profound: Inhale to prepare, exhale to move. Or, more specifically for the walking cycle: Inhale to lift and gather, exhale to step and root.

Consider the mechanics of the Tai Chi step. It involves a phase of "emptying" one leg (lifting the foot) and a phase of "filling" the other leg (placing the foot and shifting weight). The inhalation should accompany the lifting phase. As the breath is drawn in, the body naturally creates a subtle upward energy. This lightness assists in peeling the heel off the ground and suspending the leg in the air. The lungs fill, the spine lengthens, and the body gathers its resources. This is the "yin" phase of the movement—internal, gathering, and preparatory.

The exhalation coincides with the "yang" phase—the exertion and the rooting. As the foot touches the ground and the weight begins to shift onto it, the practitioner exhales. This exhalation should be slow, controlled, and typically done through the nose or through pursed lips. Breathing out facilitates a downward flow of energy. As the air leaves the lungs, the chest sinks, the shoulders drop, and the center of gravity lowers. This "sinking" sensation is crucial for stability. It physically helps to root the foot into the earth. If one were to inhale while stepping down, the energy would be rising while the foot is trying to ground, creating a conflict in the body's momentum. Exhaling while stepping aligns the pneumatic pressure with the gravitational force, making the stance solid and immovable.

This coordination creates a natural speed governor for the walk. Since the movement must match the breath, and the breath should be slow and deep, the walking pace inevitably slows down. This is a desirable outcome. Slowing down increases the time the body spends on one leg, which drastically improves balance and leg strength. It forces the practitioner to move with intention rather than momentum. A typical cycle might look like this: Inhale for a count of three while shifting weight back and lifting the front heel. Pause for a split second. Exhale for a count of four while placing the heel forward and rolling the foot flat. The exhalation is slightly longer than the inhalation to ensure the lungs are fully emptied, preventing the buildup of stale air and carbon dioxide.

There is a critical safety component to this coordination: avoiding the Valsalva maneuver. The Valsalva maneuver occurs when a person holds their breath and strains, closing the glottis. This often happens instinctively when someone is concentrating hard or exerting effort, such as trying to balance on one leg. Holding the breath increases intrathoracic pressure, which can cause a sudden spike in blood pressure followed by a rapid drop. For a senior, this fluctuation can lead to dizziness, seeing stars, or even fainting. By strictly adhering to the "exhale to move" rule, the practitioner ensures that they never hold their breath during the difficult part of the movement. Continuous breathing keeps the blood pressure stable and ensures a steady supply of oxygen to the brain, maintaining mental clarity and focus.

Integrating breath with movement transforms the walk into a moving meditation. The mind has no room to wander to worries about the future or regrets about the past; it is fully occupied with the task of matching the airflow to the footfall. This singular focus induces a "flow state," a psychological zone where the activity feels effortless and enjoyable. The walk becomes a rhythmic cycle of tension and release, gathering and expanding. It turns a mundane physical activity into a holistic exercise that trains the respiratory system and the musculoskeletal system simultaneously. The breath acts as the conductor, and the limbs are the orchestra; when they follow the baton, the result is a symphony of coordinated, graceful motion.

Using breath to manage pain flare-ups during exercise

Pain is an inevitable companion for many seniors, whether it stems from osteoarthritis, sciatica, or old injuries. However, the reaction to pain often exacerbates the suffering. The natural human instinct when feeling a twinge of discomfort is to freeze. The muscles tighten around the painful area to splint it, the breath stops, and the mind fixates on the sensation. This reaction, while protective in the short term, creates a vicious cycle. The holding of breath deprives the muscles of oxygen, causing lactic acid to build up. The tensing of muscles compresses the joints further, increasing the mechanical irritation. The mental fixation amplifies the pain signal. Breath is the most effective tool for breaking this cycle and managing pain flare-ups in real-time.

The primary technique for pain management is "breathing into the pain." This is a visualization and relaxation method. When a sensation of stiffness or ache arises—perhaps in a knee or hip—the practitioner should not stop the walk immediately (unless the pain is sharp or severe), but rather slow down and direct the breath toward that area. On the inhalation, imagine the oxygen traveling specifically to the tight joint, surrounding it with warm, healing energy. On the exhalation, visualize the tension leaving the body with the breath, like gray smoke. This visualization serves a physiological purpose: it directs the conscious mind to release the guarding tension in the muscles surrounding the joint. By consciously relaxing the quadriceps around a sore knee on the exhalation, the joint space opens slightly, reducing the grinding sensation.

Exhalation is the key to pain relief. The act of exhaling triggers a relaxation response in the skeletal muscles. Long, audible exhalations—sighing out tension—can reset the pain threshold. When a flare-up occurs, the practitioner should switch to a specific breathing pattern: inhale for a count of two, and exhale for a count of four or six. Extending the exhalation shifts the body chemistry away from acidity and towards an alkaline state, which is less conducive to inflammation. It also engages the parasympathetic nervous system, which releases natural endorphins—the body's painkillers. This chemical shift can reduce the perception of pain significantly, turning a sharp stab into a manageable dull ache that allows the exercise to continue.

Breath also provides a sense of agency and control. Chronic pain often makes individuals feel like victims of their own bodies, leading to feelings of helplessness and fear of movement (kinesiophobia). By using the breath to modulate the sensation, the practitioner regains the driver's seat. They learn that they can influence their own comfort level. Instead of reacting with fear—"Oh no, my back hurts, I must stop"—they respond with strategy—"My back is tight, I will breathe into the lumbar region and soften the muscles." This shift in mindset is empowering. It transforms the walk from a test of endurance into a dialogue with the body.

Furthermore, rhythm acts as a hypnotic analgesic. A steady, rhythmic breath entrains the brain. Just as a mother rocks a baby to soothe it, the rhythmic motion of Tai Chi walking combined with rhythmic breathing creates a soothing oscillation in the nervous system. This rhythmic input can compete with pain signals entering the spinal cord, effectively "closing the gate" on pain transmission. This is known as the Gate Control Theory of pain. The non-painful input (rhythm, breath, movement) overrides the painful input.

It is important, however, to distinguish between managing discomfort and ignoring injury. Breathing techniques are designed to manage the "rust" of arthritis and the stiffness of inactivity. They are not meant to mask acute injury. If breathing and softening do not alleviate the pain, or if the pain escalates, the activity must stop. The breath is a diagnostic tool as much as a therapeutic one. If one cannot breathe deeply and smoothly because the pain is too intense, the body is signaling that the limit has been reached. In this way, the breath acts as the ultimate safety monitor, ensuring that the practice remains healing and never harmful. By befriending the breath, the senior practitioner gains a powerful ally, one that is always available, free of charge, and capable of transforming the experience of pain into an opportunity for release and relaxation.

Chapter 5

The Art of Weight Shifting

The ability to move through the world with stability and grace is not merely a matter of muscular strength; it is fundamentally a question of weight distribution. In the practice of Tai Chi walking, the concept of weight shifting is elevated to a precise art form, distinguishing it from the often unconscious and haphazard way human beings typically ambulate. Ordinary walking is frequently described by biomechanists as "controlled falling," where the body leans forward and the legs scramble to catch the center of gravity. This method relies on momentum and allows for a dangerous moment of instability between steps. Tai Chi walking reverses this dynamic. It demands that the practitioner maintain complete control over their balance at every millisecond of the stride. This control is achieved through the meticulous separation of weight, ensuring that the body is never caught in a vulnerable middle ground. Mastering the transfer of mass from one leg to the other is the secret to moving without the fear of falling, transforming the act of walking into a continuous flow of rooted power.

"Full" vs. "Empty" Leg: Understanding how to transfer weight completely before stepping

At the heart of Tai Chi walking lies the concept of "Full" and "Empty," or in traditional terms, the distinction between substantial and insubstantial. This is the practical application of Yin and Yang theory to human locomotion. A "Full" leg is the leg that bears one hundred percent of the body's weight. It is the pillar, the foundation, and the root. It connects deeply with the earth, the muscles engaged and the joints aligned to support the entire skeletal structure. Conversely, the "Empty" leg bears zero weight. It is light, mobile, and free to move without friction or hesitation. The Empty leg is not limp or dead; it is alert and ready, but it is unburdened by the task of support. The most common error in senior mobility—and the primary cause of stumbling—is a failure to distinguish between these two states. When weight is distributed evenly, perhaps split 50/50 or 60/40 between the feet during a step, the individual is "double-weighted." In this state, neither leg is fully rooted, and neither leg is fully mobile. If a person trips while double-weighted, the leg needed to recover balance is trapped by the partial weight it is carrying, unable to move quickly enough to catch the body.

The process of shifting from Full to Empty must be absolute and deliberate, comparable to pouring water from one vessel to another. Imagine an hourglass. The sand flows from the top bulb to the bottom bulb. It does not exist in both simultaneously with equal mass. Similarly, as the practitioner prepares to take a step, the weight must pour entirely into the standing leg. Only when the standing leg is completely Full—firmly rooted, knee soft, hip settled—can the other leg become completely Empty. This emptiness allows the foot to peel off the ground effortlessly, heel first, then toe. There is no need to "heave" the leg up or use momentum to swing it forward. Because it carries no weight, the Empty leg can be placed gently and precisely, like a cat testing the ground. The foot touches down without committing weight immediately. This is a critical safety mechanism. If the foot lands on a patch of ice, a loose rug, or an uneven cobblestone, the weight has not yet been transferred. The practitioner can simply lift the Empty foot and place it somewhere safer, all while remaining securely balanced on the Full leg.

This methodology radically changes the rhythm of walking. It introduces a momentary pause, a sensation of stillness within the motion. The cycle involves filling the leg, rooting, emptying the other leg, stepping, and only then beginning the transfer of weight. This transfer must be gradual. The practitioner pushes from the Full leg, sending the center of gravity forward in a smooth horizontal line. As the weight flows into the front leg, it gradually transitions from Empty to Full. Simultaneously, the rear leg transitions from Full to Empty. There is a precise crossover point, but because the movement is controlled by the muscles rather than gravity, the practitioner remains stable throughout. This creates a sensation of gliding. The head remains at a constant level, avoiding the vertical bobbing motion characteristic of regular walking. This level movement indicates that the knees are doing their job as shock absorbers and that the weight transfer is efficient.

Sensory awareness plays a pivotal role in this practice. The practitioner must learn to feel the pressure changes in the soles of the feet. The "Bubbling Well" point, located just behind the ball of the foot, acts as the primary sensor. As the leg becomes Full, the sensation of pressure at this point intensifies, as if the foot is melting into the floor. The sensation extends upward, engaging the calf, the thigh, and the glute. The bones align—ankle, knee, and hip stack vertically to channel the force of gravity directly into the ground. If the alignment is off, the muscles must strain to hold the body up, leading to fatigue. When the alignment is true, the Full leg feels surprisingly effortless, supported by the ground reaction force. Conversely, the Empty leg should feel airy and spacious in the hip joint. By cultivating this binary awareness—heavy vs. light, rooted vs. mobile—the senior walker eliminates the ambiguity that leads to falls. The body is always somewhere definite, never lost in the chaotic transition between steps.

Developing the core strength needed to stand on one leg (even for a split second)

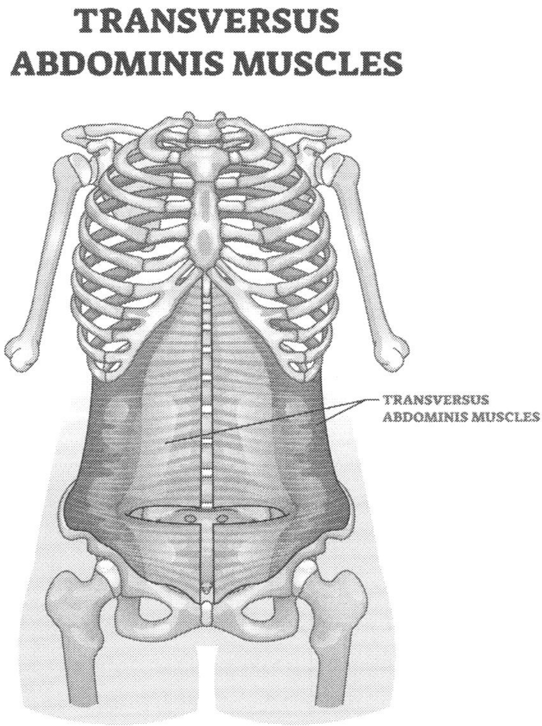

While the legs facilitate the transfer of weight, the core provides the stabilization required to maintain that weight on a single column of support. The ability to stand on one leg, even for the brief duration of a stride, is the ultimate litmus test of functional balance. In the context of Tai Chi walking, "core strength" does not refer to the superficial abdominal muscles often associated with gym culture. Instead, it refers to the deep, intrinsic stabilizers of the trunk: the transverse abdominis, the multifidus, the pelvic floor, and the psoas. These muscles form an internal cylinder that wraps around the spine and organs, providing a solid center from which the limbs can move. Without this central stability, the torso collapses or twists when the weight is shifted to one side, forcing the body to compensate by flailing the arms or taking a rapid, uncontrolled step.

The connection between the core and the single-leg stance is biomechanical. When one foot lifts off the ground, the body's base of support shrinks from a wide rectangle (two feet) to a small single point (one foot). Gravity immediately tries to pull the torso toward the unsupported side. The deep core muscles must fire instantaneously to resist this rotational force and keep the pelvis level. If the core is weak, the hip of the swinging leg drops, a phenomenon known as the Trendelenburg sign. This drop destabilizes the knee of the standing leg and throws the spine out of alignment.

Strengthening the core allows the practitioner to "lift" the torso out of the hips, creating space for the legs to move freely. This lifting action is subtle—internal rather than external—often described in Tai Chi as "suspending the spine" while "sinking the pelvis."

Developing this specific type of strength requires slow, isometric engagement rather than rapid crunches. The core must learn to hold the body still against the pull of gravity. The Dan Tian, the energy center located roughly two inches below the navel and deep inside the body, serves as the focal point for this strength. The practitioner learns to move from this center. Before lifting a leg, the intention settles in the Dan Tian. The abdominal muscles tighten slightly, not rigidly, but with the tone of a drum skin. This pre-activation braces the spine. As the weight shifts onto the Full leg, the core acts as the anchor. It prevents the upper body from leaning excessively to the side. A common mistake is to lean the shoulders far over the standing leg to maintain balance. While this works mechanically, it is precarious. True balance comes from a vertical spine supported by a strong core, allowing the weight to sink directly down through the hip rather than toppling over it.

The psoas muscle deserves special attention in this process. As the primary connector between the lumbar spine and the legs, the psoas is responsible for lifting the thigh. In many seniors, the psoas is tight and weak from prolonged sitting. When the psoas is dysfunctional, the leg feels heavy, and lifting it requires strain in the lower back. Tai Chi walking rehabilitates the psoas by demanding a gentle, controlled lift of the knee with every step. This action is powered by the core, not just the hip flexors. By visualizing the leg movement originating from the Dan Tian, the deep abdominal muscles engage to assist the lift. This integration makes the leg feel lighter and reduces the effort required to keep it in the air during the transfer phase.

Fear is a significant barrier to single-leg balance. The brain perceives the moment of lifting a foot as a threat to survival. This fear triggers tension, which paradoxically makes balance more difficult. The core strength developed in Tai Chi walking provides a physiological counter to this psychological fear. When the practitioner feels a strong, internalized corset of muscle supporting their spine, confidence grows. The "split second" of single-leg stance extends into a second, then two. The rush to put the foot down subsides. This patience is the hallmark of strength. It allows the individual to hover the empty foot, adjusting its placement if necessary, rather than stomping it down in panic. Training the core to support this hovering moment is training the body for fall prevention. It buys the brain time—time to assess the terrain, time to correct a stumble, and time to move with decision rather than reaction.

Drill: The "Tree in the Wind" weight-shift exercise

To internalize the mechanics of Full and Empty legs and to build the requisite core stability, specific drills are more effective than simply trying to walk immediately. The "Tree in the Wind" is a foundational exercise designed to isolate the lateral weight shift, slowing the process down so the mind can map the movement accurately. This drill removes the complexity of stepping, allowing the practitioner to focus entirely on the sensation of filling and emptying the legs while maintaining an upright, relaxed posture. It serves as a laboratory for balance, a safe space to experiment with the limits of stability without the risk of moving forward.

The setup for the drill is simple yet precise. The practitioner stands with feet wider than shoulder-width apart—a "Horse Stance" or Ma Bu, though a high, gentle version is sufficient. The feet are parallel, toes pointing straight ahead. The knees are unlocked, soft, and slightly bent. The spine is erect, with the head suspended and the tailbone dropping straight down, eliminating the curve in the lower back. The arms can hang loosely by the sides or float in front of the abdomen as if holding a large ball, which helps to round the back and sink the chest. The visualization is that of a great tree: the legs and pelvis are the roots and trunk, solid and immovable, while the upper body is the branches, flexible and responsive. The wind blows, shifting the tree's weight, yet the roots remain deep.

The movement begins with a shift of weight to the right. The practitioner pushes from the left foot, driving the pelvis horizontally to the right. It is crucial that the hips stay level; they should glide like a puck on an air hockey table, not dip or rise. As the weight pours into the right leg, the right knee remains aligned over the toes, never collapsing inward. The nose stays aligned with the navel, ensuring the torso moves as a single unit with the hips. The goal is to reach a point where the right leg is bearing approximately 70% to 90% of the weight, while the left leg becomes light. The left foot remains flat on the floor, maintaining contact, but the pressure eases. This is the moment to check in: Is the right glute engaged? Is the right foot rooting? Is the breath sinking?

Once the limit of the shift is reached—without straining or leaning the upper body—the movement reverses. The right leg pushes into the ground, sending the pelvis gliding back to the left. The transition should be smooth, without jerks or halts. The "wind" blows the tree to the other side. Now the left leg fills, becoming the substantial pillar, and the right leg empties. The cycle repeats, a slow, rhythmic oscillation from side to side. The pace should be meditative, perhaps five to ten seconds for a single shift. This slowness forces the stabilizing muscles of the hip and core to fire continuously, building endurance. If there are gaps in strength or balance, the slow speed will reveal them as shakes or wobbles. These tremors are merely the nervous system learning new pathways; they are signs of progress.

Common errors in this drill provide valuable feedback. A frequent mistake is "breaking" at the hip, where the upper body leans in the direction of the movement while the hips shoot out in the opposite direction. This disconnects the core and destabilizes the knee. The "Tree in the Wind" requires the nose, navel, and pubic bone to remain in a vertical line. Another error is allowing the knee of the Full leg to drift past the toes or collapse inward. This places shear force on the joint. The knee must be kept strong and stable, pointing in the same direction as the second toe. The visualization of the knee pressing slightly outward against an imaginary hand can help maintain this structural integrity.

As proficiency increases, the drill can be deepened. The stance can widen slightly, or the knees can bend a fraction more, increasing the load on the leg muscles.

The percentage of weight shift can also increase, moving from a conservative 60/40 split to a near-total 99/1 transfer, where the empty foot can actually be tapped lightly on the floor to prove its emptiness. By practicing this drill daily, the neural pathways for weight shifting become myelinated—faster and more efficient. The body learns the sensation of being 100% supported on one leg. When this feeling is transferred to walking, the fear of the single-leg phase evaporates. The "Tree in the Wind" plants the seed of stability, ensuring that when the practitioner eventually steps out into the world, they do so with the rooted confidence of an ancient oak, capable of swaying with life's currents without ever being uprooted.

Chapter 6

The Tai Chi Walk Step-by-Step

The culmination of preparation, posture, and breath work finds its expression in the act of walking itself. This is not merely a method of transportation from one point to another, but a reconstructive process for the human gait. Over years of hurried movement, the natural, fluid mechanics of walking often degrade into a series of controlled collisions with the ground. The Tai Chi walk deconstructs this habit, replacing the jarring impact of a heavy stride with a sophisticated, rolling contact that preserves the joints and conserves energy. This chapter dissects the three mechanical components that define this safe stride: the rolling action of the foot, the width of the stance, and the deliberate control of speed. Mastering these elements transforms the simple act of walking into a high-level therapeutic exercise, turning every step into a deposit in the bank of physical longevity.

The Heel-to-Toe Roll: The biomechanics of a safe stride that reduces impact

The human foot is an architectural masterpiece designed to function as a rocker, a complex lever system capable of absorbing the shock of body weight and translating it into forward motion without trauma. However, in standard modern walking, particularly when wearing thick-soled shoes, this rocker function is often bypassed. The typical gait pattern involves a "heel strike"—a sharp, forceful impact where the heel hammers into the ground. This strike sends a shockwave up the tibia, through the knee, into the hip, and eventually into the lumbar spine. Over thousands of steps per day, this repetitive micro-trauma contributes significantly to the degradation of cartilage and the onset of osteoarthritis. The Tai Chi walk eliminates this impact through the "Heel-to-Toe Roll," a technique that treats the foot not as a flat paddle, but as a curved wheel.

The movement begins with the placement of the heel. Unlike the aggressive strike of regular walking, this placement is gentle. The ankle acts as a hinge, flexing upward (dorsiflexion) to present the calcaneus (heel bone) to the ground. The contact point is crucial; it should be the center-back of the heel, not the edge. Because the leg is "Empty" (carrying no weight) at the moment of contact, the touch is feather-light. It tests the terrain. Once the heel secures a purchase on the ground, the weight transfer begins, and the foot begins its roll. This roll is not a sudden slap of the sole against the pavement. It is a gradual, articulate unraveling of the foot along the floor. The sensation is often described as peeling a sticker off a backing sheet, but in reverse. The sole of the foot makes contact sequentially: first the heel, then the arch (or the lateral edge for those with high arches), then the ball of the foot, and finally the toes.

This rolling action serves a critical biomechanical function: it increases the time over which force is applied. In physics, impulse is defined as force multiplied by time. By lengthening the time it takes for the foot to bear weight, the peak force of the impact is drastically reduced. The shock is dissipated into the muscles of the calf and the intrinsic muscles of the foot rather than being absorbed by the bones and joints. This is the difference between dropping a glass onto concrete versus dropping it onto a plush pillow. The Heel-to-Toe roll turns the ground into a pillow. As the foot rolls flat, the "Bubbling Well" point behind the ball of the foot engages, signaling the brain that the foundation is secure. Only then does the full weight of the body settle onto the leg.

The completion of the roll involves the toes. In many seniors, the toes have become passive, crammed into shoes and forgotten. In the Tai Chi walk, the toes are active participants. As the weight moves forward, the toes spread and grip the ground gently. This "grasping" action activates the arch of the foot, turning it into a spring. It provides the final push-off force. Without this engagement, the foot remains a flat block, and the walker must rely on lifting the hip to move the leg, which strains the lower back. The push-off from the toes propels the body forward smoothly, utilizing the elastic energy stored in the Achilles tendon.

Developing this roll requires restoring flexibility to the ankle joint. A stiff ankle forces the foot to slap down or necessitates a shorter, shuffling stride. The practice of lifting the toe high before planting the heel stretches the calf muscle and mobilizes the ankle. This action pumps the venous blood from the lower legs back up to the heart, aiding circulation and reducing swelling in the ankles. The mental focus during the roll should be on the sensation of the ground texture. By paying attention to how the heel, arch, ball, and toes interact with the floor, the practitioner heightens proprioception. This sensory feedback loop is the body's natural defense against tripping; a foot that feels the ground is a foot that can react to it. The Heel-to-Toe roll transforms the foot from a passive hoof into an intelligent sensor, navigating the world with sensitivity and precision.

Tracking Width: Keeping feet shoulder-width apart to widen your base of support

While the Heel-to-Toe roll addresses how the foot lands, "Tracking Width" addresses where it lands. A pervasive error in the gait of aging adults—and indeed many people of all ages—is the tendency to narrow the stance. This is often a subconscious attempt to conserve energy or mimic the aesthetic of runway models who walk with one foot directly in front of the other. This "tightrope walking" style is biomechanically disastrous for stability. When the feet land in a single line, the base of support is extremely narrow laterally. The body becomes like a bicycle: stable when moving fast, but incredibly unstable when moving slow or standing still. Any lateral force—a gust of wind, a bump from a passerby, or an uneven paving stone—can easily topple the structure because there is no width to resist the tipping motion.

The Tai Chi walk corrects this by establishing a "Railroad Track" gait. The practitioner visualizes two parallel rails running along the ground, separated by the width of the shoulders or the hips. The left foot travels strictly along the left rail, and the right foot travels along the right rail. The space between the feet remains constant throughout the stride. This width creates a rectangular base of support rather than a linear one. A table with four legs spread wide is harder to tip over than a table with legs clustered in the center. By maintaining this shoulder-width spacing, the center of gravity has a much larger area in which to move safely. If the body sways to the side, the wide-set foot acts as an outrigger, catching the weight and preventing a fall.

Maintaining this width requires the engagement of the hip abductor muscles, specifically the gluteus medius. These muscles are responsible for moving the leg away from the midline. In many seniors, these muscles are atrophied due to inactivity. When the abductors are weak, the legs tend to drift inward, leading to a scissoring gait where the feet almost cross over each other. This scissoring increases the risk of tripping over one's own feet. Consciously stepping "out" as well as "forward" reactivates these critical hip stabilizers. The sensation initially may feel like waddling or walking like a cowboy. This is a common perception, but a mirror check usually reveals that what feels like a wide waddle is actually a normal, vertical anatomical alignment. The hip, knee, and ankle should form a straight vertical column.

The challenge of tracking width is most apparent during the weight shift. When walking on a tightrope, the weight transfer is minimal because the feet are already under the center. When walking on railroad tracks, the weight must travel a significant distance from the left rail to the right rail. This demands a complete lateral shift of the pelvis. The practitioner must trust the standing leg enough to move the entire torso over it before stepping out with the other leg. If the shift is incomplete, the body "falls" toward the gap between the legs, leading to instability. The wide track forces the walker to commit fully to each step, eradicating the tentative, half-hearted movements that lead to stumbles.

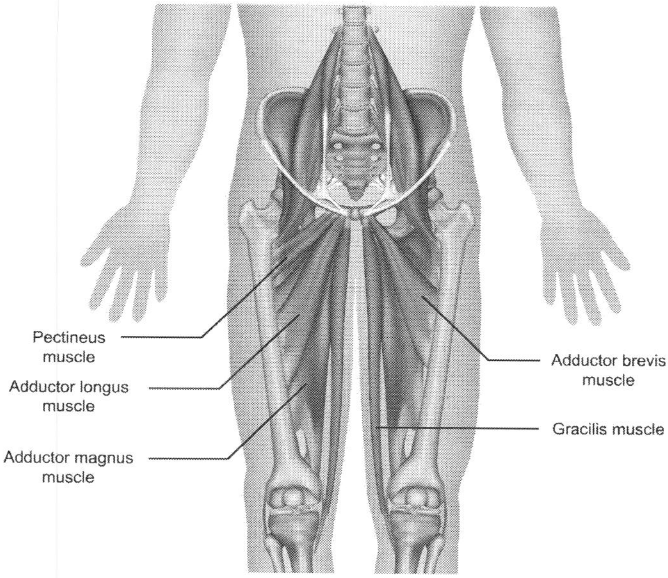

Practicing this width can be aided by visual cues. Walking along a tiled floor where the tiles form a grid is an excellent exercise; the practitioner can ensure that each foot stays in its respective lane of tiles, never encroaching on the center line. In an outdoor setting, a path with wheel ruts or a marked lane can serve the same purpose. The mental cue is "open hips." By keeping the inguinal crease (the fold of the groin) open and spacious, the legs naturally fall into a wider track. This opening also decompresses the hip joints, which can become impinged by a chronically narrow stance.

The benefits of the Railroad Track stance extend to the lower back. A narrow gait forces the pelvis to twist excessively with each step to swing the leg around. This torque places shear stress on the sacroiliac joints and the lumbar discs. A wide track allows the pelvis to remain relatively square to the front, reducing the rotational strain on the spine. The movement becomes a forward glide rather than a twisting grind. For a senior concerned with back pain, simply widening the step can offer immediate relief. It provides a stable platform for the spine to rest upon. The wider base represents a physical claiming of space; it is a posture of confidence and solidity, declaring that the walker is grounded, stable, and difficult to uproot.

Speed Control: Why slowing down actually builds muscle faster than speeding up

The final component of the Tai Chi walk is the element that most distinguishes it from Western exercise philosophy: the deliberate reduction of speed. In a culture that equates speed with fitness and intensity with results, the instruction to "slow down" can seem counterintuitive. The common assumption is that walking faster raises the heart rate and burns more calories, therefore constituting a "better" workout. However, for the purposes of balance, stability, and functional strength, speed is often the enemy. Fast movement allows the practitioner to rely on momentum. Momentum is a force that carries the body through a range of motion without the muscles having to do the work. When a person swings their leg forward quickly, inertia does the lifting. The muscles simply initiate the swing and then relax.

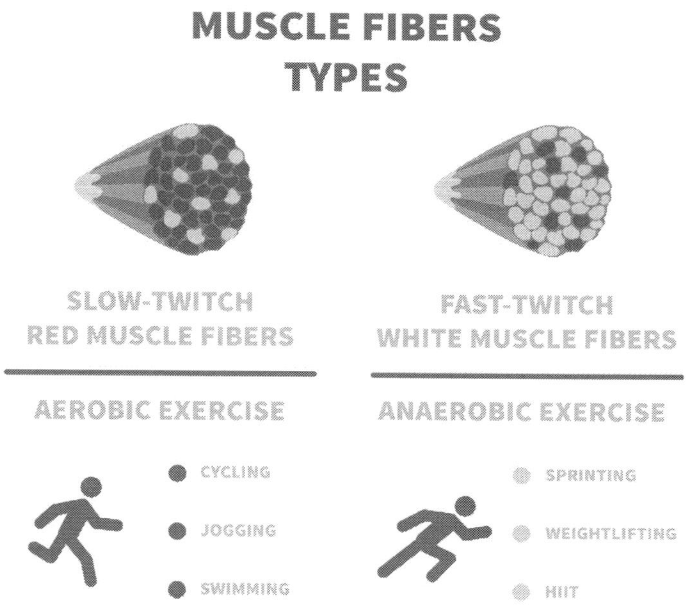

Tai Chi walking removes momentum from the equation. By slowing the movement down to a crawl—taking perhaps three to five seconds to complete a single step—the practitioner forces the muscles to engage throughout the entire trajectory of the motion. This concept is known in strength training as "Time Under Tension" (TUT). When a muscle is kept under tension for a longer duration, more muscle fibers are recruited to sustain the load. The slow-twitch fibers, which are responsible for endurance and posture, are fully activated. As they fatigue, the body begins to recruit fast-twitch fibers to assist. This results in a deeper, more comprehensive strengthening effect than rapid, momentum-driven movement. A slow, controlled step demands that the quadriceps, hamstrings, glutes, and calves work continuously to stabilize the joints against gravity.

This slow pace is particularly effective for strengthening the stabilizer muscles—the small, deep muscles around the ankle, knee, and hip that are often bypassed during fast movement. When walking quickly, the large prime movers (like the rectus femoris) take over, masking weaknesses in the smaller stabilizers. When moving slowly, any instability or weakness is immediately exposed. The leg might shake or wobble. This shaking is not a sign of failure; it is the neurological process of the brain mapping the connection to these dormant muscles. It is the sound of the body learning. By persevering through the slowness, the practitioner builds a corset of strength around the vulnerable joints, providing internal bracing that protects against injury.

Neurologically, slow movement provides the brain with the time it needs to process sensory data. As we age, the processing speed of the brain can slow down. A rapid stride might outpace the brain's ability to interpret feedback from the feet and eyes. If a slip occurs at high speed, the brain may not register it in time to send a corrective signal to the muscles. By walking slowly, the feedback loop is synchronized. The brain has ample time to feel the heel strike, sense the weight shift, and adjust the center of gravity. This "mindfulness in motion" rewires the neural pathways governing balance. It updates the body schema—the brain's internal map of where the limbs are in space. Over time, this improved mapping translates to faster reaction times even when moving at normal speeds.

The discipline of slowness also addresses the psychological "rush" that leads to falls. Many accidents occur because the mind is projected forward—thinking about the ringing phone, the boiling kettle, or the destination—while the body rushes to catch up. This disconnect creates a forward lean and a hurried, stumbling gait. Practicing Tai Chi walking requires a conscious braking of this impulse. It teaches the practitioner to inhabit the present step fully before moving to the next. This mental discipline of "arriving before leaving" bleeds into daily life. The practitioner learns to pause before standing, to turn slowly, and to walk with deliberate intent.

Achieving this slowness requires a continuous, fluid engagement, like moving through water. The resistance of the air should be visualized as the resistance of water, requiring a steady, hydraulic push. There should be no stops or starts, just a continuous, uniform velocity. This smooth deceleration creates a unique aesthetic and feeling of control. It turns the walk into a power stance. The heart rate may not spike as high as it does during a jog, but the muscular fatigue will be evident. The legs will burn, the core will tighten, and the body will generate heat. This is the "internal work" or Nei Kung. It builds a density of muscle and a resilience of tendon that light, fast aerobics cannot replicate. By slowing down, the senior walker is not regressing; they are engaging a higher gear of biomechanical efficiency, building the kind of functional strength that holds the body upright for a lifetime.

PART 3

TARGETED SOLUTIONS – JOINTS AND FALLS

Chapter 7

Soothing the Joints (Knees, Hips, and Ankles)

For the aging body, the joints often serve as the loudest barometer of health, signaling the weather changes, the level of previous exertion, and the passage of time with a language of creaks, stiffness, and aches. It is a common misconception that joint pain is a command to stop moving. In reality, stillness is often the enemy of joint health. The cartilage that cushions the bones relies entirely on movement for its survival and repair. However, not all movement is created equal. High-impact activity can degrade fragile surfaces, while aimless motion may fail to stimulate the necessary healing responses. The Tai Chi method offers a precise, medicinal approach to movement, utilizing specific biomechanical principles to nourish the knees, hips, and ankles. This chapter demystifies the biology of joint lubrication and provides a roadmap for modifying these powerful movements to accommodate arthritis and surgical replacements, ensuring that the practice remains a source of relief rather than a cause of distress.

Why low-impact rotation lubricates the joints (synovial fluid explained simply)

To understand why Tai Chi walking is so effective for joint relief, one must first understand the unique anatomy of the joint itself. Unlike muscles, skin, or organs, the articular cartilage—the smooth, white coating on the ends of bones—is avascular. It has no blood supply. It cannot receive oxygen or nutrients from the heart's pumping action. Instead, it relies on a specialized substance called synovial fluid. This fluid is the body's internal motor oil, a thick, egg-white-like substance rich in hyaluronic acid and lubricin. Its primary function is to reduce friction, allowing bones to glide over one another seamlessly. However, its secondary function is nutritional. Synovial fluid carries the essential nutrients the cartilage needs to stay spongy and resilient.

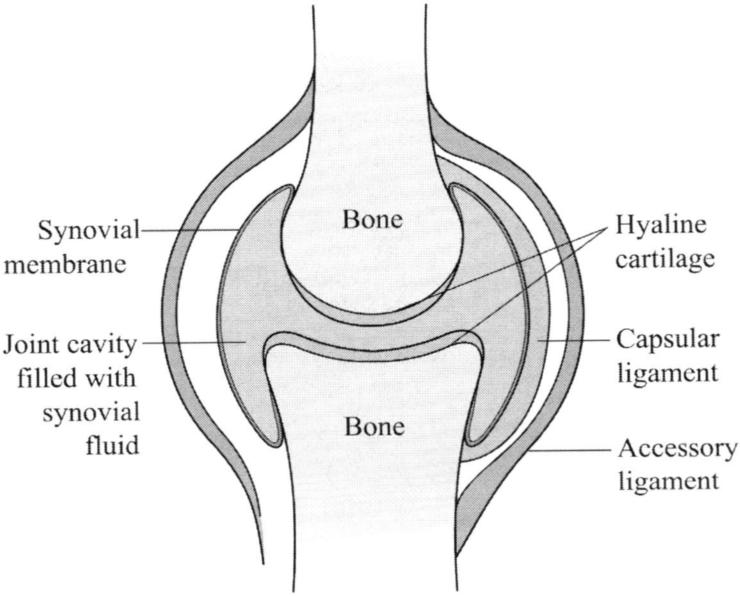

The delivery mechanism for these nutrients is a process known as imbibition, which functions remarkably like a sponge in water. When a joint bears weight, the cartilage is compressed, and waste products are squeezed out. When the weight is removed or the joint is opened, the pressure releases, and the cartilage sucks in fresh, nutrient-rich synovial fluid. This cycle of compression and release is the heartbeat of joint health. If a person sits all day, the sponge remains stagnant; it dries out, becomes brittle, and begins to decay. This is why morning stiffness is so prevalent—the joints have been immobile for hours. Conversely, pounding the pavement with heavy steps is like hitting the sponge with a hammer; it damages the structure before it can absorb fluid. Tai Chi walking hits the "Goldilocks" zone: rhythmic, gentle loading that pumps the fluid without crushing the matrix.

Rotation adds a critical dimension to this process. Most daily movements—walking to the fridge, climbing stairs, standing up—are linear. They occur in the sagittal plane, moving strictly forward and backward. This linear movement utilizes only a small track of the joint surface, wearing it down over time like a tire that is never rotated. The rest of the cartilage remains underutilized and under-nourished. Tai Chi walking incorporates subtle, internal spirals and rotations. As the weight shifts and the waist turns, the ball of the femur rotates gently within the hip socket. This rotational action smears the synovial fluid across the entire surface area of the joint capsule, reaching the "corners" that linear walking misses. It ensures that the entire cartilage surface is bathed in nutrients.

Furthermore, the "low-impact" nature of the movement is key to stimulating the synovial membrane. This membrane, which lines the joint capsule, produces the fluid. Research suggests that gentle, repetitive motion stimulates the membrane to secrete more fluid and to improve the viscosity of that fluid. When a joint is inflamed or arthritic, the fluid can become thin and watery, providing less protection. The slow, controlled compression of Tai Chi walking encourages the production of thicker, more protective fluid. It acts as a hydraulic buffer. By moving slowly, the practitioner allows the fluid to distribute evenly, creating a hydro-dynamic film that separates the bones. This implies that the bones are literally floating on a layer of liquid, rather than grinding against each other.

The concept of "Song"—or conscious relaxation—during movement plays a vital physiological role here. When muscles around a joint are tense (a common reaction to pain), they compress the joint space, increasing friction. By actively relaxing the quadriceps and hamstrings during the Empty phase of the step, the joint space opens up. This distinct phase of "opening" creates a vacuum effect, drawing fluid into the deepest layers of the cartilage. Therefore, the Tai Chi step is a pump: step down to squeeze out waste, lift and relax to soak in nutrients. Repeating this cycle thousands of times during a walk provides a massive dose of therapeutic lubrication, often resulting in joints that feel warmer, looser, and less painful at the end of the walk than they did at the start.

Modifications for those with arthritis or previous joint replacements

While the principles of Tai Chi walking are universally beneficial, the application must be customized for those navigating the specific challenges of osteoarthritis, rheumatoid arthritis, or total joint arthroplasty (replacements). The standard advice to "listen to the body" is insufficient here; specific mechanical adjustments are required to ensure safety and prevent the aggravation of existing conditions. For the practitioner with arthritis, the primary adversary is bone-on-bone friction. When the protective cartilage has worn away, the grinding sensation can be debilitating. The most important modification in this scenario is the reduction of the range of motion (ROM) to stay strictly within the "pain-free envelope."

For knee osteoarthritis, deep knee bends are often the trigger for sharp pain. The traditional Tai Chi instruction to "sink low" must be discarded in favor of a "high stance." The practitioner should keep the knees relatively straight, maintaining only the "soft" unlock described in earlier chapters. The degree of flexion might be only five or ten degrees. This minimizes the sheer force on the patella and the tibiofemoral joint while still allowing for the weight-shifting mechanics to function. Additionally, the stride length should be shortened significantly. A long stride requires the lead leg to extend fully and the heel to strike with more force. By taking smaller steps—perhaps only half the length of a normal stride—the foot can land flatter and softer, reducing the impact shock that travels to the damaged knee.

For those with hip replacements, particularly recent ones, adhering to medical precautions is paramount. The risk of dislocation, though low in modern prosthetics, is highest when the leg is internally rotated and adducted (crossed over the midline) simultaneously. Therefore, the "Tracking Width" discussed in Chapter 6 becomes a non-negotiable safety rail. The practitioner must ensure the feet never cross the center line. The stance should be wider than usual to provide stability without risking impingement. Furthermore, when turning, the turn must originate from the feet, not the torque of the hip. Instead of planting the foot and twisting the body (which grinds the hip), the practitioner should pick up the foot and reposition it in the direction of the turn. This "step-turn" technique protects the prosthetic interface.

Ankle stiffness or fusion requires a different approach. If the ankle cannot dorsiflex (bend upward) sufficiently, the Heel-to-Toe roll becomes difficult. Forcing it can cause the knee to hyperextend. In such cases, the modification is to adopt a "flat-footed" placement. The practitioner places the entire foot down gently at once, like a stamp.

To compensate for the lack of ankle roll, the knees must be extra soft to absorb the landing. The focus shifts from the rolling of the foot to the fluidity of the weight transfer. The goal remains the same—smooth, impact-free movement—but the mechanism is adapted to the available hardware.

Rheumatoid arthritis (RA) presents a variable challenge, as symptoms fluctuate with flare-ups. During an active flare, when joints are hot, swollen, and red, the intensity of the practice must be dialed down to near zero. The "walk" may become a seated practice, visualizing the steps and performing gentle, non-weight-bearing oscillations of the legs to keep fluid moving without stress. Pushing through the inflammation of an RA flare can damage the joint capsule. Conversely, during remission, it is vital to gently expand the range of motion to prevent the formation of scar tissue and contractures. The use of assistive devices should be destigmatized in this context. Using walking poles (Nordic walking sticks) can offload up to 30% of the weight from the lower body, transferring it to the arms and core. This allows the arthritic senior to practice the Tai Chi gait with proper form and duration, gaining the cardiovascular benefits without punishing the knees.

Psychological modification is equally important. Those with chronic joint pain often develop "guarding" patterns—holding the breath and tensing the body in anticipation of pain. This tension acts as a corset, compressing the joints further. The practice must involve a conscious "un-guarding." Before every movement, a mental scan is performed to release the grimace in the face, the shrug in the shoulders, and the grip in the glutes. The mantra for the arthritic practitioner is "smoothness over depth." It does not matter how low the stance is or how long the stride is; if the movement is jerky, it is harmful. If it is smooth, continuous, and connected to the breath, it is healing, regardless of how small the external movement appears.

Movements to loosen stiffness in the morning vs. cooling down at night

The circadian rhythm of the joints dictates that the body requires different mechanical inputs at different times of the day. A routine that feels miraculous at 6:00 PM might feel impossible or even damaging at 7:00 AM. Understanding the physiological state of the tissues upon waking versus their state before sleep allows the practitioner to tailor the practice for maximum efficacy, turning the daily cycle into a loop of preparation and recovery.

In the morning, the body is in a state of "cold stiffness." During the night, body temperature drops, blood flow to the extremities decreases, and the intervertebral discs hydrate and swell, making the spine feel stiff and inflexible. The synovial fluid in the peripheral joints has settled and become more viscous, like cold honey. The primary goal of the morning routine is mobilization and heat generation. It is about melting the honey. Static stretching—holding a position for a long time—is generally contraindicated immediately upon waking, as cold tissues are prone to tearing. Instead, the focus should be on dynamic, oscillatory movements.

A highly effective morning sequence begins even before leaving the bed. "Bed cycling" involves lying on the back and gently pedaling the legs in the air. This removes gravity from the equation, allowing the knees and hips to move through their range of motion without load. It pumps old fluid out and pulls new fluid in. Upon standing, the "Tai Chi Swing" is the gold standard for waking up the spine. The practitioner stands with feet wide, knees soft, and arms loose. The movement is a gentle rotation of the waist from left to right, allowing the arms to flop heavily against the body like empty coat sleeves. This rotational force gently wrings out the stiffness in the back muscles and stimulates blood flow to the kidneys and adrenal glands. The emphasis is on rhythm and looseness, not stretching.

Another vital morning movement is "Ankle Circling." Standing on one leg (with support), the practitioner rotates the free ankle in slow, deliberate circles, first clockwise, then counter-clockwise. This is crucial because stiff ankles force the knees and hips to compensate during the first steps of the day. By mobilizing the ankles first, the entire kinetic chain is prepped for a proper gait. The morning session should be characterized by "Yang" energy—rising, active, and warming. The breathing should be slightly more vigorous to oxygenate the blood and wake up the nervous system.

Normal Venous Return

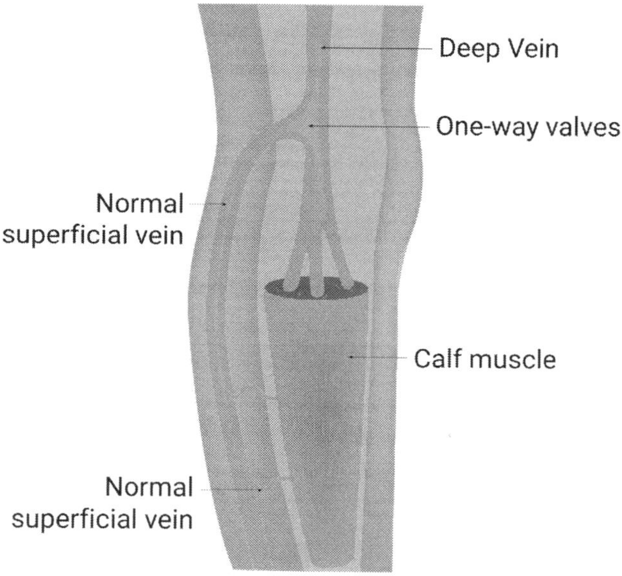

In contrast, the evening physiology is characterized by compression and fatigue. After a day of upright activity, gravity has compressed the spinal discs and the cartilage in the knees and hips. Fluids may have pooled in the lower legs (edema), causing swollen ankles. The muscles may be short and tight from overuse. The goal of the evening routine is decompression and drainage. It is about "Yin" energy—sinking, cooling, and restoring.

Dynamic, bouncy movements should be avoided as they can overstimulate the nervous system before sleep.

The "Golden Rooster Stands on One Leg" is an excellent evening posture, provided it is done with support. By standing still on one leg for 30 to 60 seconds (switching sides), the practitioner forces the blood to return from the feet to the core, aiding venous return and reducing swelling. The focus here is not on the struggle to balance, but on the "sinking" sensation, allowing gravity to pull the tension out of the shoulders and hips. Following this, the "Supported Spine Hang" (a modified forward fold with hands on a kitchen counter or table) allows the lumbar spine to traction gently. The practitioner walks the feet back and leans forward, keeping the back flat, letting the weight of the hips pull backward. This creates space between the vertebrae, counteracting the day's compression.

In addition, the evening routine should conclude with "breathing into the joints." In a seated or lying position, the practitioner performs a body scan. Locating areas of heat or throbbing (common in arthritic joints after a long day), they use the exhalation technique discussed in Chapter 4. They visualize cool, blue light entering the joint, soothing the inflammation. Gentle, slow-motion flexion and extension of the toes and fingers can help dissipate residual tension. The evening practice is not about building muscle; it is about resetting the baseline tone of the nervous system so that the body can enter deep sleep, which is the only time true tissue repair takes place. By respecting this duality—mobilizing the cold stiff body and soothing the hot tired body—the practitioner ensures that the cycle of mobility is sustainable day after day.

Chapter 8

Fall-Proofing Your Life

Proprioception: Retraining your brain to know where your feet are without looking

The human body possesses a sophisticated internal navigation system that operates entirely below the level of conscious thought. While sight, sound, and touch are the celebrated senses, a hidden sixth sense known as proprioception serves as the silent guardian of stability. Proprioception is the continuous feedback loop between the sensory receptors in the joints, muscles, and skin, and the central nervous system. It tells the brain exactly where the body is positioned in space, the angle of the ankle, the bend of the knee, and the texture of the ground, all without the need for visual confirmation. In youth, this system is lightning-fast and accurate. However, the aging process often dulls these signals. Nerve conduction velocity slows down, and the receptors in the feet—mechanoreceptors—become less sensitive. Consequently, the brain receives a "fuzzy" map of the body's position. To compensate for this loss of internal data, many seniors unconsciously develop a dependency on vision. They begin to look down at their feet while walking to confirm where they are stepping.

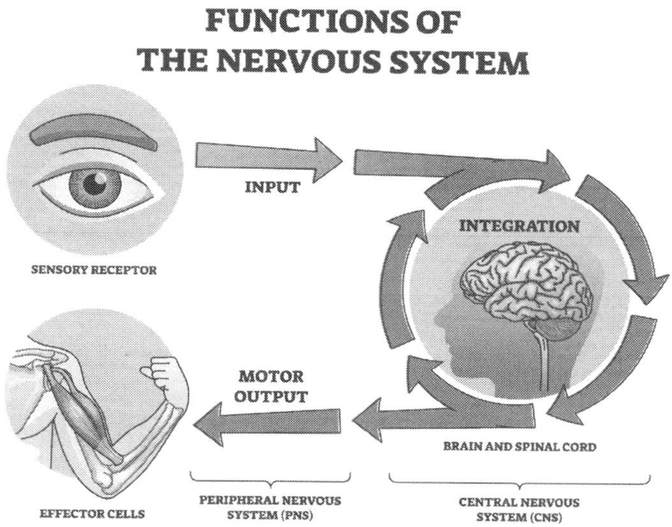

This visual dependency creates a perilous biomechanical trap. When the head drops to look at the ground, the heavy weight of the skull pulls the cervical spine forward. This shifts the body's center of gravity anteriorly, placing the individual in a perpetual state of falling forward. Furthermore, relying on vision means the brain is reacting to the environment rather than sensing it. Visual processing is slower than tactile processing. By the time the eyes register an uneven paving stone and the brain commands the leg to adjust, the stumble may have already occurred. Retraining proprioception involves breaking this visual addiction and waking up the dormant sensors in the lower limbs. The goal is to shift the reliance from the eyes back to the "feeling" intelligence of the body.

The process of retraining begins by removing the visual input in a controlled, safe environment. Standing near a sturdy counter or wall for safety, the practitioner closes their eyes. Immediately, the body may begin to sway. This sway is not a failure; it is the brain frantically searching for data. Without the horizon line to lock onto, the brain is forced to listen to the ankles and the soles of the feet. This heightened demand strengthens the neural pathways. The practitioner focuses intensely on the "Bubbling Well" point on the sole of the foot and the pressure distribution across the heel and toes. Even thirty seconds of "blind standing" daily acts as a high-intensity workout for the vestibular and proprioceptive systems. As confidence grows, the exercise can advance to shifting weight from side to side with eyes closed, further challenging the internal gyroscope.

Another powerful method for sharpening this sense is the exploration of texture. Modern life creates a sensory vacuum for the feet, as thick rubber soles and flat floors provide very little feedback. To counteract this, the practitioner can practice walking barefoot or in thin socks on varied surfaces within the home—shifting from the hardness of tile to the softness of carpet, or stepping onto a foam mat. This variety forces the mechanoreceptors to fire in different patterns, refreshing the neural map. The conscious mind must engage with these sensations. Instead of ignoring the feeling of the floor, the individual actively interrogates it: Is this surface hard or yielding? Is it slippery or grippy? Is it cold or warm? This mindful inquiry amplifies the signal volume traveling from the foot to the brain.

The ultimate aim of proprioceptive training is to allow the gaze to return to the horizon. When the brain trusts the feet to navigate the micro-terrain, the eyes are freed to scan the macro-environment—looking for traffic, obstacles, or changing weather conditions. This "heads-up" posture keeps the spine vertical and the center of gravity strictly over the base of support. It restores the natural dignity of the gait. A walker who looks ahead projects confidence and awareness, while a walker who looks down projects fear and vulnerability. By systematically retraining the brain to feel the earth, the senior practitioner builds a foundation of safety that functions in the dark, in crowds, and in complex environments where vision alone is insufficient.

Recovery steps: What to do if you feel a stumble coming on

Despite the best preparation and the strongest proprioception, the unpredictable nature of the world means that stumbles can still occur. A hidden root, a patch of black ice, or a sudden jostle in a crowd can disrupt equilibrium. In these critical milliseconds, the difference between a harmless stumble and a catastrophic hip fracture lies in the body's automated reaction. For the untrained individual, the instinctive response to a loss of balance is the "startle reflex." This primitive survival mechanism causes the body to stiffen, the breath to freeze, and the arms to flail upwards. While this might ward off a predator, it is disastrous for gravity. Stiffening the legs raises the center of gravity and turns the body into a rigid toppling tree. The flailing arms disconnect the core stabilizers. To fall-proof the life, one must overwrite this startle reflex with a trained "recovery reflex."

The core principle of a safe recovery is "Sinking." The moment instability is felt—that sickening lurch of the stomach—the trained response is to immediately drop the center of gravity. This is achieved by bending the knees and exhaling sharply. Biomechanically, lowering the hips brings the body closer to the ground, increasing stability and reducing the potential distance of a fall. It transforms the body from a top-heavy inverted pendulum into a stable pyramid. The exhalation is crucial because it releases the tension in the diaphragm and the psoas, preventing the rigid locking of the torso. This "drop" buys the brain a fraction of a second to deploy the legs for a rescue maneuver.

The primary physical tool for catching a fall is the "Recovery Step" or the "Lunge Step." Unlike the timid, shuffling steps often taken by fearful walkers, a recovery step must be dynamic, wide, and explosive. If the body begins to tip to the right, the right leg must shoot out aggressively to the side—wider than the shoulder—to create a new base of support that catches the falling weight. The error most people make is stepping too narrow or crossing the legs. If the recovery step crosses the midline, it creates a tripping hazard against the other leg. The Tai Chi training of "Tracking Width" discussed in previous chapters ingrains the habit of keeping the legs in their respective lanes. In a stumble, this training ensures the leg shoots out to an open space, acting as an outrigger.

Once the recovery foot hits the ground, it must do so with a "stomp" or a firm plant, immediately followed by the "soft knee" absorption. If the recovery leg lands locked straight, the momentum of the fall will vault over it, continuing the topple. If the knee bends upon impact, it acts as a shock absorber, dissipating the kinetic energy of the stumble. The muscles of the thigh (quadriceps) must perform a strong eccentric contraction—lengthening under load—to brake the movement. This is why the slow, strengthening drills of the Tai Chi walk are so vital; they build the specific leg strength required to arrest the weight of the falling torso.

Practicing these recovery strategies requires a safe environment, ideally with a spotter or in a pool where the water supports the weight. The practitioner can deliberately induce small imbalances—leaning slightly too far forward or to the side—and practice the "Sink and Step" response. The mental cue is "Down and Out": drop the hips down, step the foot out. By rehearsing this scenario, the brain creates a motor program that can fire faster than conscious thought. Instead of freezing in panic, the body activates a practiced subroutine. It turns a potential emergency into a managed event. The stumble becomes a "stutter step," a brief interruption in rhythm rather than a life-altering accident. This active defense system empowers the senior to move through the world not with the fragility of glass, but with the resilience of rubber, ready to bounce back from the unexpected.

Navigating uneven terrain: Applying Tai Chi walking on grass, gravel, and slopes

The sterile, flat environment of a hallway or a gym is the classroom, but the chaotic, textured surface of the real world is the exam. Nature rarely offers perfectly level ground. Grass hides dips and divots; gravel creates a rolling, unstable surface; and slopes alter the physics of every step. To maintain independence, the Tai Chi walker must adapt the fundamental principles of the stride to conquer these variable terrains. The key adaptation is a shift from the rhythmic, rolling gait used on flat ground to a more tactile, probing, and conservative methodology suitable for the wild.

Walking on grass or soft earth presents a unique challenge because the ground absorbs energy. The rebound force that usually helps propel the walker forward on pavement is lost in the soil. Furthermore, the visual uniformity of a lawn can mask holes or exposed roots. The adaptation here is the "High Stepping" variation of the Tai Chi walk. The practitioner must lift the knee slightly higher than usual, ensuring the foot clears the top of the grass blades and any potential hidden obstacles. The placement of the foot changes from a heel-roll to a flatter, more tentative placement. The foot hovers for a split second before committing weight, "listening" to the ground to ensure it is solid. If the foot senses a hole or a rock, the weight remains on the back leg, and the foot is repositioned. This requires significant single-leg balance, reinforcing the need for the core strength developed in earlier chapters.

Gravel or loose stones act like ball bearings underfoot. A long stride with a heavy heel strike on gravel creates a shearing force that can cause the foot to slide forward, leading to a backward fall. To navigate this, the stride length must be drastically shortened. The foot should be placed down as vertically as possible, minimizing the forward slide. The practitioner imagines they are walking on a sheet of ice. The entire sole of the foot contacts the gravel almost simultaneously, trapping the stones underneath rather than pushing them away. The weight transfer must be delayed until the foot is fully planted and the stones have "settled" under the load. The center of gravity is kept lower than usual, with the knees bent more deeply to lower the body's pivot point.

Slopes, particularly stepping downhill, are the nemesis of the aging joint. Going downhill places immense pressure on the knees and requires the braking strength of the quadriceps. The instinct is to lean back away from the slope, but this is dangerous as it positions the center of gravity behind the heels, inviting a slip that results in the feet flying out forward. The counter-intuitive correct technique is to keep the torso perpendicular to the slope—or even leaning slightly forward—keeping the weight over the center of the foot. The knees must remain perpetually bent, never straightening fully. This "Groucho Marx" style of walking keeps the muscles engaged and protects the knee joints from snapping back.

For steep inclines, whether up or down, the "Zig-Zag" strategy is the ultimate energy saver and safety tactic. Walking straight up or down the fall line of a hill requires maximum ankle flexibility and strength. By traversing the slope diagonally, the effective gradient is reduced. The practitioner walks across the face of the hill, turns 180 degrees (using a safe, wide turn), and walks back across. This switchback pattern reduces the angle of the ankle and provides a more stable platform for the foot. On the uphill phase, the focus is on driving from the glutes, pushing the ground away. In the downhill phase, the focus is on "yielding" to gravity, stepping softly and silently.

Navigating uneven terrain is as much a psychological challenge as a physical one. It requires the suppression of the "rush" impulse. When faced with a rough patch of ground, the natural tendency is to hurry across it to get back to safety. The Tai Chi approach is the opposite: the rougher the ground, the slower the movement. The practitioner enters a state of hyper-awareness, treating the terrain as a puzzle to be solved one step at a time. The gaze scans continuously, mapping the path three or four steps ahead. By mastering these surfaces, the world expands. The practitioner is no longer confined to the shopping mall or the sidewalk but is free to explore the garden, the woodland path, and the beach. The uneven ground ceases to be a threat and becomes a training partner, constantly challenging and refining the balance that preserves freedom.

PART 4

INTEGRATION – MAKING IT A HABIT

Chapter 9

Building Your Daily Routine

The transformation from a person who struggles with balance to a person who moves with fluid confidence does not occur in a single dramatic session of exertion. It occurs in the quiet, consistent accumulation of small moments. The grandest intentions often crumble under the weight of a rigid, hour-long gym schedule, but micro-habits—movements woven seamlessly into the fabric of daily life—have the power to endure. The goal of this final section is to dismantle the idea that exercise must be a separate event, divorced from the rest of the day. Instead, the principles of Tai Chi walking are integrated into the mundane activities of brewing coffee, sitting on a park bench, or navigating the first month of practice. By anchoring these movements to existing triggers, the practice ceases to be a chore and becomes a natural, sustaining rhythm of life.

The "5-Minute Coffee Break" routine

The morning kitchen offers a perfect, often overlooked sanctuary for balance training. The period spent waiting for the kettle to boil or the coffee to brew provides a distinct, consistent window of time that can be reclaimed for physical cultivation. This "dead time," usually spent staring blankly or scrolling through a phone, is transformed into a ritual of awakening the nervous system. The environment is ideal: the kitchen counter is typically the perfect height to serve as a stability bar, offering a sturdy, waist-high support that allows for safe experimentation with balance before the brain is fully alert. This routine begins the moment the button on the machine is pressed.

The first movement in this sequence is the "Counter-Supported Weight Shift." Standing facing the counter, with hands resting lightly on the edge, the individual adopts the shoulder-width stance discussed in earlier chapters. The objective is not to walk, but to wake up the feet. Slowly, the weight is poured entirely into the left leg until the right foot becomes "empty." The heel of the empty foot lifts slightly, hovering for a second, before rolling back down. The weight then pours slowly into the right leg, freeing the left. This oscillation mimics the slow rhythm of the coffee dripping. The hands on the counter provide a safety net, allowing the practitioner to close their eyes and focus entirely on the internal sensation of pressure changing in the soles of the feet. This simple shifting pumps fluid into the stiff morning knees and hips, lubricating the joints before the demands of the day begin.

As the steam begins to rise, the routine transitions to "Heel Peels." Still holding the counter, the practitioner keeps both toes on the ground and alternately lifts one heel and then the other, as if pedaling a bicycle in slow motion. This action stretches the plantar fascia—the connective tissue on the bottom of the foot that often becomes tight and painful overnight (plantar fasciitis). It also pumps venous blood from the lower legs back up to the heart, combating any swelling that may have settled during sleep. The movement should be rhythmic and gentle, synchronized with deep, diaphragmatic breaths. Inhaling as a heel rises, exhaling as it sinks. This synchronization links the breath to the movement, calming any morning anxiety and setting a tone of deliberate focus for the day ahead.

The final minute of the brew cycle is dedicated to the "Teacup Squat." This is a functional strengthening exercise disguised as a stretch. Holding the counter firmly, the practitioner keeps the spine vertical—head suspended, tailbone tucked—and slowly bends the knees, lowering the hips straight down as if sliding the back against a wall. The depth is minimal, perhaps only two or three inches. The focus is on keeping the knees soft and aligned over the toes, avoiding the tendency for them to collapse inward. This mini-squat engages the quadriceps and the glutes, the primary anti-gravity muscles. Holding the position for a count of five while breathing deeply builds isometric strength. Upon rising, the legs push the floor away, straightening without locking the knees. By the time the coffee is ready, the body has been scanned, lubricated, and activated. This five-minute ritual requires no change of clothes and no equipment, yet it ensures that the first movements of the day are mindful and stable, rather than stiff and reactive.

The "Park Bench" workout

Venturing outdoors adds the variables of fresh air, visual stimulation, and social interaction, all of which are vital for holistic health. However, the prospect of a long walk can be daunting for a beginner. The "Park Bench" workout reframes the outdoor experience. The bench is not merely a place to rest when exhausted; it is a piece of gym equipment, a destination, and a safety station all in one. By centering the workout around a bench, the fear of fatigue is mitigated. The practitioner knows that a seat is always within arm's reach, which psychologically permits them to push their limits slightly further than they might on an open path.

The core of this routine is the "Sit-to-Stand" repetition, arguably the single most important exercise for maintaining independence in old age. The ability to rise from a chair without using hands is the primary indicator of leg strength and functional longevity. The park bench, often slightly lower than a standard dining chair, offers a challenging height. The exercise begins by scooting to the front edge of the bench, feet planted firmly at shoulder width. The critical mechanic here is the "Nose Over Toes" lean. To rise efficiently, the upper body must hinge forward at the hips until the nose is vertically aligned over the toes. This shifts the center of gravity forward, allowing the legs to drive the body upward. The practitioner exhales and pushes the earth away, rising to a full stand, then slowly—taking three full seconds—lowers back down. Gravity is resisted on the way down; collapsing into the seat is avoided. Performing five to ten of these repetitions builds massive power in the thighs and hips.

Once the legs are warm, the bench serves as a support for standing balance drills. Moving to the back of the bench (or the side if it has no back), the practitioner places hands on the backrest. This solid support allows for the practice of "Hip Abduction." Standing on one leg, the other leg is lifted slowly out to the side, keeping the toes pointed forward. This targets the gluteus medius, the muscle responsible for pelvic stability and preventing the "waddle" gait. Weakness in this muscle is a leading cause of falls. The bench provides the security needed to perform this movement without the risk of toppling over.

The movement is small and controlled, focusing on the squeeze in the outer hip rather than the height of the leg.

The bench also facilitates a safe stretch for the hamstrings and calves, which are often tight in seniors. Standing facing the bench, one foot is placed on the seat (or the lower rail if the seat is too high). With a soft standing knee and a tall spine, the practitioner hinges forward slightly from the hips, keeping the back flat. This creates a gentle stretch along the back of the raised leg. Stretching in the park offers a dual benefit: the physical release of tension and the mental release of "forest bathing." While holding the stretch, the gaze can take in the trees, the sky, and the horizon, engaging the peripheral vision which is linked to the parasympathetic nervous system. This creates a state of relaxed alertness.

The workout concludes with "Mindful Observation." Sitting back on the bench, the practitioner engages in a period of active recovery. This is not checking a phone or rumination. It is a conscious practice of diaphragmatic breathing while observing the environment. Watching people walk by becomes a study in biomechanics—noticing who rushes, who leans forward, who walks with fluidity. This observation reinforces the learning from the book. By identifying the "falling forward" gait in others, the practitioner reinforces their own commitment to the Tai Chi principles of vertical alignment and weight separation. The park bench becomes a classroom, and the workout ends not with exhaustion, but with a sense of connection to the community and the natural world.

Structuring a 4-week progression plan for absolute beginners

Ambition is a powerful engine, but without a steering wheel, it can drive a beginner off the road. The most common error in starting a mobility practice is doing too much, too soon. The soft tissues—tendons and ligaments—adapt much slower than muscles or enthusiasm. To build a habit that lasts, the intensity must be titrated carefully. A four-week progression plan serves as a scaffold, ensuring that the foundation is cured before weight is added to the structure. This plan prioritizes consistency over duration, and quality over quantity.

Week 1: The Awakening. The first week is dedicated entirely to awareness and static mechanics. There is no pressure to "go for a walk" in the traditional sense. The goal is simply to inhabit the body. The daily requirement is ten to fifteen minutes, split into micro-sessions. The focus is on the "internal scan." The practitioner spends this week mastering the posture: suspending the head, sinking the chest, and softening the knees. The exercises are performed primarily in the kitchen or living room. The "**Coffee Break**" routine is established here. The primary metric of success in Week 1 is not distance covered, but the frequency of "checking in." How many times a day did the individual notice their shoulders were tense and drop them? How many times did they correct their posture while brushing their teeth? This week re-calibrates the proprioceptive system.

Week 2: The Shift. As the body becomes comfortable with the static posture, the second week introduces the dynamic of weight transfer. The focus shifts to the concept of "**Full and Empty**." The daily practice extends to twenty minutes. The specific drill for this week is the "**Tree in the Wind**" exercise **(Chapter 5)** and the "**Counter-Supported Weight Shift**." The practitioner learns to separate the weight completely before lifting a foot. This is the week of slow-motion drills. Walking is performed only in a hallway or a clear room, taking perhaps only ten steps back and forth, but taking them with excruciating slowness. The goal is to eliminate the wobble. If a wobble occurs, the practitioner stops, resets, and starts again. This week builds the core stability required for single-leg balance.

Week 3: The Stride. With the vertical alignment and weight shifting mechanics installed, the third week integrates the footwork. This is the week of the

"**Heel-to-Toe Roll**." The practice moves to the "**Railroad Track**" width. The practitioner begins to take short walks outside—perhaps just to the mailbox or the end of the driveway. The focus is on the sensory feedback from the feet. The practitioner actively focuses on the heel striking gently, the foot rolling flat, and the toes pushing off. The duration increases to twenty-five minutes, but the pace remains deliberately slow. This is the "testing phase" where the mechanics meet the friction of the real world (shoes, pavement, uneven concrete). The "**Park Bench**" workout components can be introduced here, specifically the sit-to-stand strength work.

Week 4: The Flow. The final week of the introductory month is about synthesis. The separated elements—posture, shift, and step—are smoothed into a continuous rhythm. The breath is synchronized with the movement (inhale to lift, exhale to step). The duration extends to thirty minutes of continuous movement. This is where the practice transforms from a set of drills into a "walk." The practitioner ventures further—around the block or through the park loop. The mental cue shifts from specific mechanics to a general sense of "flow." The walk should feel liquid and connected. If pain or fatigue arises, the practitioner reverts immediately to the Week 1 principles of relaxation. Week 4 is the launchpad. By the end of this month, the habit is no longer a foreign imposition; it is a familiar friend. The neural pathways have been blazed, the joints have been lubricated, and the fear of falling has been replaced by a toolkit of recovery and strength. The journey has officially begun.

Conclusion

Moving Forward with Confidence

Recap of the journey

The path traveled through the pages of this guide mirrors the physical journey of the Tai Chi walker: it begins with a pause, establishes a root, and then proceeds with deliberate, mindful intention. At the outset, the concept of walking was likely viewed through the lens of utility—a means of getting from the bedroom to the kitchen, or from the car to the store. For many, this simple act had become fraught with a quiet, underlying tension, a subtle fear of the ground rising up to meet them. The transformation that has occurred is not merely a collection of exercises, but a fundamental reconstruction of the relationship with gravity. The journey began by challenging the pervasive myth that a loss of balance is an inevitable tax of aging. It established that the body, regardless of its chronological age, retains a remarkable plasticity. The muscles can learn new firing patterns, the nervous system can sharpen its proprioceptive map, and the skeleton can rediscover its vertical alignment. This realization is the bedrock upon which all subsequent techniques were built.

The foundation was laid in the preparation of the physical vessel. The assessment phase stripped away the assumptions of capability and replaced them with objective data about range of motion and stability. By identifying the "danger zones" in the home and the habits of the body, the practitioner moved from a state of unconscious vulnerability to one of conscious awareness. The seemingly mundane act of choosing the correct footwear was revealed to be a critical safety decision, turning the shoe from a fashion statement into a piece of precision equipment that facilitates sensory feedback. The environment itself was transformed from an obstacle course into a dojo, a sanctuary where the floor is cleared and the lighting is optimized to support the work of balance.

From this safe space, the pillars of posture were erected. The instruction to "suspend the head" acted as the vertical plumb line, organizing the spine and relieving the compressive burden of gravity. Sinking the chest and raising the back moved the center of calm to the solar plexus, replacing the anxious, high-chest breathing of the startle reflex with the deep, diaphragmatic respiration of the master. The softening of the knees became the secret to shock absorption, turning rigid stilts into responsive springs capable of navigating a hard world without shattering. These static principles were then animated by the engine of breath. The synchronization of inhalation with preparation and exhalation with movement created a physiological rhythm that calmed the nervous system, proving that stability is as much a state of mind as it is a state of muscle.

The mechanics of the movement—the core of the Tai Chi stride—dismantled the habit of "controlled falling." The distinction between the "Full" and "Empty" leg revolutionized the transfer of weight. No longer was the body caught in the dangerous limbo of being double-weighted; instead, it learned the discipline of pouring weight completely into one rooted leg before risking the movement of the other. The Heel-to-Toe roll replaced the jarring impact of the heel strike with a smooth, articulate interaction with the ground, turning every step into a massage for the joints. Tracking width provided the lateral stability of a railroad car, preventing the scissoring gait that leads to trips. Finally, the deliberate reduction of speed—the embrace of slowness—built the deep, intrinsic strength that momentum had previously masked.

This technical proficiency was then applied to the specific challenges of the aging body. The joints, often sources of pain and limitation, were reimagined as sponges needing the rhythmic compression of movement to stay lubricated. The modifications for arthritis and joint replacements ensured that the practice remained inclusive, proving that pain does not dictate the end of mobility, only the need for adaptation. The fall-proofing strategies—proprioceptive training and the recovery step—provided an insurance policy, a set of emergency protocols ingrained in the muscles to handle the unexpected. By the time the daily routine was established, the practice had shifted from a series of disjointed drills into a cohesive lifestyle. The coffee break, the park bench, and the hallway became opportunities for cultivation. The journey has not been linear; it has been a spiral, circling back to the same principles of relaxation and root with ever-increasing depth and understanding. The walker who stands at the end of this book is not the same person who opened it. They are grounded, they are aware, and they possess the tools to navigate the world with a dignity that commands space.

Invitation to view walking as a meditation

The physical benefits of Tai Chi walking—stronger legs, better balance, reduced pain—are profound, yet they are merely the external manifestation of an internal shift. To view walking solely as a biomechanical exercise is to miss the deeper invitation it offers: the opportunity to turn a mundane daily necessity into a profound meditative practice. Meditation is often misunderstood as the act of sitting in a pretzel shape, trying to empty the mind of all thought. This static definition can feel inaccessible or frustrating to those with active minds or aching bodies. Tai Chi walking offers an alternative: meditation in motion. It anchors the wandering mind not to a mantra, but to the visceral reality of sensation. The mind cannot be worrying about the future or regretting the past when it is fully occupied with the complex task of peeling the heel, rolling the arch, and grasping with the toes.

This practice transforms the sidewalk into a sanctuary. In the rush of modern life, the body is often treated as a vehicle to transport the head from one meeting to another. The mind projects forward to the destination—the grocery store, the doctor's office, the mailbox—leaving the body to trail behind, hurried and unnoticed. This disconnection is the root of anxiety. Tai Chi walking reunites the mind and body in the present moment. By focusing on the breath—inhaling to gather, exhaling to root—the practitioner enters a state of flow. The chatter of the "monkey mind" quiets down, replaced by the rhythmic feedback of the foot against the earth. This is the state of "Sung," or conscious relaxation, where the body is alert but not tense, moving with the fluidity of water.

Walking thus becomes a dialogue with the environment. Instead of tuning out the world with headphones or internal rumination, the senses are dialed up. The proprioceptive system feels the subtle incline of the pavement; the ears hear the rhythm of the breath; the eyes scan the horizon with a soft, panoramic gaze. This heightened awareness is the essence of mindfulness. It changes the quality of the experience. A walk to the mailbox is no longer a chore to be rushed through; it becomes a few minutes of self-care, a check-in with the self. "How is my posture today? Am I holding tension in my shoulders? Can I sink my weight a little deeper?" These questions bring the individual back to the "now," the only place where life actually happens.

This meditative approach also reframes the relationship with pain and limitation. In a standard exercise mindset, pain is an obstacle to be conquered or ignored. In a meditative mindset, sensation is simply information. If a knee feels stiff, the meditative walker does not judge it or force it; they acknowledge it, breathe into it, and adjust the movement to accommodate it. There is a compassion in this approach. It fosters a friendship with the body rather than a dictatorship. The walk becomes a daily act of gratitude for what the body can do, rather than a lament for what it can no longer do. This shift in perspective reduces the cortisol levels associated with stress and pain, creating a biochemical environment that supports healing.

Furthermore, viewing walking as meditation infuses the day with pockets of peace. One does not need to carve out an hour for a yoga class to find tranquility. The thirty seconds it takes to walk from the living room to the kitchen can be a meditation. The walk from the car to the pharmacy entrance can be a practice of grounding. By stringing these pearls of mindfulness together, the entire day is elevated. The frantic, rushing energy that leads to falls is replaced by a deliberate, calm cadence. The practitioner learns to move through the world with the majestic slowness of a ship entering a harbor, fully in control, fully present. This presence projects an energy of stability that others can feel. It is a reclaiming of dignity. To walk with meditation is to declare that the journey is just as important as the destination, and that every step is an opportunity to arrive home in one's own body.

Encouragement to join a community or find a walking buddy

While the internal work of Tai Chi walking is a solitary endeavor, the maintenance of the habit thrives on connection. The path to wellness can sometimes feel lonely, especially when facing the unique challenges of aging. Pain and the fear of falling can be isolating forces, keeping individuals confined to their homes, shrinking their world to the four walls of safety. Breaking this isolation is as vital for health as the exercises themselves. The final step in mastering this art is to bring it out of the living room and into the community. Humans are inherently social creatures, wired for connection. When movement is shared, it becomes sustainable, enjoyable, and deeply reinforcing.

Finding a walking buddy transforms the practice from a discipline into a date. Accountability is a powerful motivator. on days when the weather is gray or the joints are stiff, the knowledge that a friend is waiting at the park bench provides the necessary nudge to put on shoes and step out the door. This partnership creates a safety net. Walking with a companion reduces the anxiety of navigating uneven terrain or venturing further from home. There is a "safety in numbers" effect that allows the nervous system to relax more deeply than when walking alone. Furthermore, a buddy serves as a mirror. They can offer gentle feedback—"You're leaning forward a bit," or "Your shoulders look tense"—helping to correct form that the practitioner might not feel internally.

Beyond the practical benefits, the social component of walking stimulates the brain. Conversation requires cognitive processing—listening, formulating responses, recalling memories—all while navigating the physical environment. This "dual-tasking" is the gold standard for cognitive health, warding off decline and keeping the mind sharp. However, with Tai Chi walking, the conversation takes on a different quality. It is not the breathless gossip of a power walk; it is the paced, rhythmic exchange that matches the stride. There is room for silence, for shared observation of nature, for a connection that goes beyond words.

If a single partner is unavailable, joining or forming a community group can be transformative. Across the world, parks are filled with groups practicing Tai Chi and walking arts. These "Sanghas" or communities offer a sense of belonging. Seeing others—some perhaps older or with more physical challenges—moving with grace and confidence is incredibly inspiring. It provides proof of concept. It normalizes the struggle and celebrates the progress. The collective energy of a group moving in unison creates a powerful field of focus that uplifts the individual practice. It is harder to quit when one is part of a team.

For those who have mastered the basics outlined in this book, there is an invitation to lead. Teaching is the highest form of learning. One does not need to be a grandmaster to show a friend how to do the "Heel-to-Toe Roll" or how to "Sink the Chest." Sharing these tools with a spouse, a neighbor, or a grandchild reinforces the knowledge and provides a service to the community. It creates a ripple effect of stability. Imagine a neighborhood where the seniors walk not with fragility, but with the grounded power of the Tai Chi stride, looking out for one another, moving together.

Ultimately, the goal is to integrate this new way of moving into the fabric of social life. Instead of meeting for coffee and sitting, meet for a "Tai Chi stroll." Make the walk the social event. By linking the physical practice with emotional connection, the habit becomes unbreakable. The fear of falling is replaced by the joy of participation. The world opens up again. The park, the museum, the city street—these are no longer forbidden zones, but playgrounds. The journey does not end with the last page of this book; it continues in every step taken with intention, in every breath shared with a friend, and in the quiet confidence of knowing that the ground is no longer an enemy, but a firm and supporting friend.

Printed in Dunstable, United Kingdom

81050318R10069